The Mediterranean Diet Decoded

Your Comprehensive Guide to Achieving Optimal Health, Weight Loss, and Anti-Aging Benefit

Betty B. Burton

Table of Contents

Introduction

In the hustle and bustle of modern life, where the relentless pace often leaves us gasping for a moment of respite, our health can unintentionally become the casualty of our ambitions. Picture this: You're on the treadmill of life, chasing deadlines, and juggling responsibilities, and somewhere in the frenzy, the essence of well-being slips through the cracks.

I've been there.
I know the struggle of glancing in the mirror and wondering, "Is this the best version of myself?" It's the internal dialogue we all engage in, wrestling with the desire for optimal health, sustainable weight loss, and that elusive secret to aging gracefully.

Enter the Mediterranean Diet.
This is not just a diet; it's a journey, a voyage back to the roots of wholesome living. As I dove into the Mediterranean lifestyle, I uncovered not just a guide to eating but a roadmap to transforming my entire well-being. The discoveries were so profound, so game-changing, that I felt compelled to share them with you.

In these pages, we'll decode the mysteries of the Mediterranean Diet together. It's not about deprivation or unrealistic promises; it's about embracing a lifestyle that celebrates the joy of eating, nourishing your body with foods that resonate with centuries of wisdom, and reclaiming the vitality that often eludes us in the chaos of the modern world.

So, if you're tired of fad diets that promise the moon but deliver only disappointment if you're yearning for a holistic approach to health that feels more like a lifelong companion than a temporary fix, then join me on this transformative journey.

Let's decode the Mediterranean Diet and rediscover the incredible potential within ourselves to achieve optimal health, weight loss, and a life rich with anti-aging benefits. Your journey to a healthier, happier you begins now.

Chapter 1

Understanding the Basics

Principles of the Mediterranean Diet

In the realm of diets, where trends rise and fall like waves, there's one that has weathered the storms and emerged as a beacon of longevity, flavor, and vitality, the Mediterranean Diet. As we embark on this journey to understand its principles, envision a lifestyle that transcends the restrictive norms of traditional diets, inviting you to savor not just your food but every moment of your life.

At the heart of the sun-kissed shores of the Mediterranean lies a secret, a lifestyle that has sustained generations, fostering health, resilience, and a profound connection to the pleasures of nourishment. The Mediterranean Diet isn't a fleeting solution; it's a tapestry woven with the threads of tradition, science, and the simple joy of eating well.

Principles of the Mediterranean Diet:

1. Abundance of Fresh, Colorful Produce:

Imagine your plate as a canvas, adorned with the vibrant hues of nature. The Mediterranean Diet champions a rich tapestry of fruits, vegetables, and herbs, delivering a symphony of flavors and a spectrum of essential nutrients.

2. Heart-Healthy Fats, Especially Olive Oil:

Bid farewell to the misconception that all fats are foes. Embrace the golden elixir of the Mediterranean, olive oil. Its heart-protective properties and rich taste are a testament to the diet's celebration of wholesome, unprocessed fats.

3. Lean Proteins, Primarily Fish and Legumes:

Picture a seaside feast featuring succulent fish and hearty legumes. The Mediterranean Diet emphasizes lean protein sources that not only satiate but also contribute to sustained energy and muscle health.

4. Whole Grains as the Foundation:

Imagine the hearty aroma of whole grains filling your kitchen. The diet places whole grains at its core, offering a steady release of energy and a robust foundation for overall well-being.

5. Moderate Consumption of Dairy and Red Wine:

Raise a toast to moderation. The Mediterranean Diet allows for the enjoyment of dairy in moderation and, for those who appreciate it, a glass of red wine, an embodiment of the diet's holistic approach to pleasure and balance.

6. Herbs and Spices as Flavorful Allies:

Picture a pinch of oregano, a dash of thyme, and the fragrance of garlic infusing your dishes. The diet's reliance on herbs and spices not only elevates taste but also adds a healthful dimension, showcasing the marriage of flavor and well-being.

Why it Works:

The magic of the Mediterranean Diet lies not in deprivation but in abundance. It embraces the notion that food is not just fuel but a celebration, an integral part of the human experience. The diet's principles, rooted in simplicity and authenticity, offer a realistic and sustainable path to optimal health, weight management, and a joyous connection with your body.

Your Actionable Step:

As we delve deeper into this chapter, consider this your invitation to reimagine your plate. Take a moment to envision a meal that not only nourishes your body but also satisfies your soul. The journey begins with understanding the basics, and the basics begin with a commitment to a lifestyle that transcends the ordinary, a commitment to the Mediterranean way. Are you ready to embrace it?

Key Components of the Diet

As we unravel the layers of the Mediterranean Diet, envision a culinary journey where taste isn't sacrificed for health, and nourishment is a celebration. In this chapter, we dive into the key components that transform a meal into a masterpiece, fostering not only well-being but a love affair with food.

The Mediterranean Triad: Olive Oil, Grains, and Fresh Produce

1. Olive Oil: Liquid Gold of the Mediterranean:

Picture the golden glow of olive oil cascading over a salad or infusing warmth into a dish. A cornerstone of the diet, olive oil is more than a culinary indulgence, it's a health elixir. Packed with monounsaturated fats and antioxidants, it's the key to heart health and longevity.

2. Whole Grains: The Steady Foundation:

Imagine a table adorned with hearty whole grains, farro, quinoa, and bulgur. These grains not only anchor your meals with satisfying robustness but also provide a slow-release energy source, keeping you fueled throughout the day.

3. Abundance of Fresh Fruits and Vegetables:

Envision a plate bursting with colors, crisp greens, succulent tomatoes, and the jewel tones of berries. The Mediterranean Diet is synonymous with a rich tapestry of fresh produce, delivering a myriad of vitamins, minerals, and phytonutrients essential for vitality.

Protein Harmony: Seafood, Legumes, and Lean Meats

4. Seafood: Ocean's Bounty for Heart Health:

Picture a seaside feast featuring grilled fish and seafood paella. The diet's emphasis on fatty fish like salmon and sardines provides a rich source of omega-3 fatty acids, promoting cardiovascular health and cognitive function.

5. Legumes: Humble Powerhouses of Nutrition:

Imagine a bowl of velvety hummus or a hearty lentil soup. Legumes, from chickpeas to lentils, form a crucial protein source in the Mediterranean Diet, offering fiber, vitamins, and minerals while contributing to sustained energy.

6. Lean Meats in Moderation:

Picture a Mediterranean gathering with a modest portion of lean meats, grilled to perfection. While the diet leans towards plant-based proteins, it allows for the enjoyment of lean meats in moderation, ensuring a balance of nutrients and flavors.

Dairy, Nuts, and the Elegance of Moderation
7. Moderate Dairy Consumption:

Envision a dollop of Greek yogurt or a sliver of feta enhancing your dishes. The Mediterranean Diet advocates for moderate consumption of dairy, providing calcium for bone health and adding a creamy touch to meals.

8. Nuts and Seeds: Nature's Nutrient-Rich Gems:

Picture a sprinkle of almonds on your morning yogurt or a handful of walnuts for an afternoon snack. Nuts and seeds, rich in healthy fats, protein, and antioxidants, offer a delightful crunch and a nutritional boost.

Balancing Act: Red Wine, Herbs, and Spices
9. Red Wine: A Toast to Moderation:

Imagine a leisurely evening, a glass of red wine in hand. In moderation, red wine becomes not just a beverage but a part of the Mediterranean Diet's philosophy, enjoyment in moderation, with potential heart health benefits.

10. Herbs and Spices: Culinary Alchemy for Health:
Picture the aroma of rosemary-infused roasted vegetables or the warmth of cinnamon in a dessert. Herbs and spices not only elevate the taste but also contribute to the diet's health benefits, offering a treasure trove of antioxidants and anti-inflammatory compounds.

Your Flavorful Journey:
As we navigate through these key components, consider this chapter a guide to assembling your Mediterranean palette. Embrace the art of combining these elements, creating meals that not only nourish your body but also tantalize your taste buds. The Mediterranean Diet isn't just about eating; it's about savoring, a symphony of flavors that resonate with health, happiness, and the simple joy of living well. Are you ready to infuse your life with this flavorful essence?

Science Behind the Diet's Effectiveness

In the ever-evolving landscape of nutrition, where trends flicker like shooting stars, the enduring brilliance of the Mediterranean Diet shines through. This chapter delves into the scientific foundations that underpin its effectiveness, revealing not just a diet but a holistic approach to well-being validated by research, endorsed by experts, and embraced by those seeking a path to vitality.

Harnessing the Power of Antioxidants:

1. Polyphenols and Antioxidants: Guardians of Cellular Health:

Imagine your body as a fortress, guarded by the mighty shield of polyphenols. Abundant in fruits, vegetables, and olive oil, these compounds combat oxidative stress, fortifying your cells against the ravages of time and environmental factors.

2. Omega-3 Fatty Acids: Nourishing the Brain and Heart:

Picture omega-3 fatty acids as the elixir for your brain and heart. Abundant in fatty fish like salmon and mackerel, these essential fats not only support cognitive function but also promote cardiovascular health, reducing the risk of heart disease.

Balancing Blood Sugar and Sustained Energy:

3. Complex Carbohydrates and Fiber: Stabilizing Blood Sugar:

Envision a steady stream of energy throughout your day, courtesy of complex carbohydrates and fiber. Whole grains and legumes, integral to the Mediterranean Diet, provide a slow release of glucose, preventing spikes and crashes in blood sugar levels.

4. Healthy Fats and Weight Management:

Picture healthy fats as allies in your weight management journey. The monounsaturated fats in olive oil and the omega-3s in fish contribute to satiety, helping control appetite and promoting a healthy balance in body weight.

Inflammation: The Silent Culprit and the Diet's Defense

5. Anti-Inflammatory Properties: Taming the Flames Within:

Imagine inflammation as a silent fire within your body, and the Mediterranean Diet as the cool breeze that extinguishes it. Rich in anti-inflammatory foods like fruits, vegetables, and fish, the diet mitigates chronic inflammation, a key player in various diseases.

Heart Health and Beyond:

6. Cardiovascular Benefits: A Symphony for the Heart:

Picture a heart pulsating with vitality, fortified by the Mediterranean Diet's impact on cholesterol levels, blood pressure, and overall cardiovascular health. The diet's positive effects on heart health have been substantiated by a plethora of scientific studies.

7. Cognitive Well-Being: Nourishing the Mind:

Envision a mind that remains sharp and agile through the years. The Mediterranean Diet, with its emphasis on omega-3s, antioxidants, and anti-inflammatory foods, emerges as a safeguard against cognitive decline, promoting mental acuity and resilience.

Your Journey into Scientific Wellness:

As we traverse the scientific landscape of the Mediterranean Diet, consider this chapter your compass, a guide to the evidence-based principles that elevate this lifestyle beyond a trend. The diet isn't just a prescription for health; it's a testament to the harmony between tradition and modern science, a chorus of flavors that resonate with the very essence of a well-lived life. Are you ready to embark on a journey where science and taste converge for your holistic well-being?

Chapter 2

The Health Benefits

Cardiovascular Health

In the rhythm of life, our hearts beat as the unwavering drum, orchestrating vitality and sustaining our very existence. This chapter explores a cornerstone of the Mediterranean Diet's prowess, the profound impact it has on cardiovascular health. Picture a symphony where each nutrient, each bite, is a note that resonates with the harmonious melody of a robust, resilient heart.

The Mediterranean Symphony for Your Heart:
1. Heart-Friendly Fats: The Overture of Olive Oil:
Envision your heart as the maestro of your well-being, and olive oil as the opening notes of a heart-healthy symphony. Abundant in monounsaturated fats and antioxidants, olive oil plays a key role in lowering LDL cholesterol levels and reducing the risk of atherosclerosis and heart disease.

2. Omega-3 Fatty Acids: The Melody of Fish and Nuts:

Picture omega-3 fatty acids as the soothing cadence in your cardiovascular score. Found in fatty fish like salmon, as well as nuts and seeds, these essential fats regulate blood pressure, decrease inflammation, and contribute to overall heart health.

Blood Pressure Harmony:

### 3.	Potassium-Rich	Foods:	Regulating	the Cardiovascular Beat:

Imagine potassium as the conductor, orchestrating the ebb and flow of your blood pressure. The Mediterranean Diet, rich in fruits, vegetables, and legumes, provides ample potassium, promoting a healthy balance and reducing the risk of hypertension.

4. Reducing Inflammatory Crescendos:

Envision inflammation as the dissonant notes in your cardiovascular symphony. The anti-inflammatory nature of the Mediterranean Diet, with its abundance of fruits, vegetables, and olive oil, acts as a soothing balm, mitigating chronic inflammation and safeguarding your heart.

Cholesterol Mastery:

5. Fiber and Whole Grains: Cleansing the Cardiovascular Score:

Picture fiber as the cleansing breeze in your cardiovascular melody. Whole grains, a staple of the Mediterranean Diet, lower cholesterol levels, sweep away excess fats and contribute to a healthy cardiovascular profile.

Your Heart's Encore:

As we journey through the intricacies of cardiovascular health in the Mediterranean Diet, let this chapter be a crescendo, a call to action for your heart's encore. Picture a life where your heart beats not just in existence but in exuberance, where each nutrient-laden bite is a standing ovation to a heart that thrives. Are you ready to let the Mediterranean Diet compose a symphony of cardiovascular vitality in your life?

Weight Management

In the kaleidoscope of well-being, weight management is a delicate dance, a dance where the Mediterranean Diet takes center stage, guiding you towards a balanced and sustainable lifestyle. Picture a journey where weight isn't just shed; it's gracefully and naturally balanced, reflecting the principles of a diet that cherishes both health and pleasure.

Balancing Act:

1. Healthy Fats and Satiety:

Envision a table adorned with the golden glow of olive oil, a feast that not only delights the palate but also fosters a sense of satisfaction. The healthy monounsaturated fats in olive oil contribute to a feeling of fullness, curbing unnecessary cravings and supporting a balanced caloric intake.

2. Lean Proteins for Sustained Energy:

Picture a meal featuring lean proteins, grilled fish, legumes, and a medley of vegetables. These proteins, integral to the Mediterranean Diet, not only fuel your body but also provide a sustained release of energy, preventing energy crashes and mindless snacking.

Whole Grains: The Foundation of Satiety:

3. Complex Carbohydrates for Long-Lasting Fullness:

Imagine a plate brimming with whole grains—farro, quinoa, and brown rice. These complex carbohydrates, a staple in the Mediterranean Diet, release energy gradually, keeping you full for longer periods and reducing the likelihood of overeating.

The Mediterranean Lifestyle: Mindful Eating and Pleasure in Moderation:

4. Mindful Eating Practices: Savoring Every Bite:

Envision a moment of pure indulgence as you savor each bite, the flavors unfolding on your tongue. The Mediterranean Diet encourages mindful eating, fostering a deeper connection with your food and promoting satisfaction with smaller portions.

5. Moderation: The Elegance of Controlled Pleasure:

Picture a table set with a moderate serving of your favorite dish, a balance of enjoyment and restraint. The diet's emphasis on moderation allows you to relish your favorite foods without guilt, contributing to a sustainable and enjoyable approach to weight management.

Physical Activity and the Mediterranean Lifestyle:

6. Integration of Physical Activity: A Vital Partner:

Imagine the Mediterranean landscape, the azure sea, olive groves, and people engaged in physical activity as a part of daily life. The diet isn't just about food; it's a lifestyle that integrates movement, promoting not only weight management but overall well-being.

Your Balanced Finale:

As we pirouette through the principles of weight management in the Mediterranean Diet, consider this chapter a choreography, a guide to a lifestyle where weight isn't the sole focus, but rather a natural outcome of a holistic approach to health. Picture a body that reflects not just the absence of excess weight but the presence of vitality, balance, and a profound connection with the joy of living. Are you ready to dance with the Mediterranean Diet towards a balanced and vibrant you?

Diabetes Prevention and Management

In the tapestry of health, diabetes can be a disruptive thread, yet the Mediterranean Diet emerges as a gentle yet powerful needle, weaving a pattern of prevention and management. Picture a landscape where blood sugar levels ebb and flow harmoniously, guided by the principles of a diet that values not just taste but the delicate equilibrium of well-being.

Balancing Blood Sugar:

1. Complex Carbohydrates: The Gentle Wave of Sustained Energy:

Envision a meal where whole grains, such as brown rice or quinoa, take center stage. These complex carbohydrates release glucose slowly, preventing sudden spikes in blood sugar levels and offering a steady stream of energy.

2. Fiber-Rich Fruits and Vegetables: Nourishing Stability:

Picture a plate adorned with a rainbow of vegetables and fruits. These fiber-rich gems, integral to the Mediterranean Diet, not only provide essential nutrients but also slow down the absorption of sugar, promoting stable blood sugar levels.

The Magic of Healthy Fats:

3. Monounsaturated Fats in Olive Oil: A Guardian Against Insulin Resistance:

Imagine olive oil as a shield against insulin resistance, a key factor in diabetes. The monounsaturated fats in olive oil enhance insulin sensitivity, aiding the body in utilizing glucose effectively and maintaining blood sugar balance.

4. Omega-3 Fatty Acids: The Balancing Act:

Envision a plate featuring fatty fish like salmon or trout. The omega-3 fatty acids in these fish not only contribute to cardiovascular health but also play a role in improving insulin sensitivity and supporting diabetes prevention and management.

Physical Activity and Weight Management:

5. Physical Activity as a Regulator:

Picture a walk along the Mediterranean shores, the rhythmic motion contributing to overall well-being. Physical activity, a part of the Mediterranean lifestyle, aids in weight management, enhances insulin sensitivity and contributes to balanced blood sugar levels.

6. Weight Management: A Pillar of Diabetes Care:

Envision the Mediterranean Diet as a sculptor, molding not just your diet but your weight. Maintaining a healthy weight is a fundamental aspect of diabetes prevention and management, and the diet's balanced approach supports this endeavor.

Antioxidants and Anti-Inflammatory Magic:

7. Antioxidants and Anti-Inflammatory Foods: Protecting Against Complications:

Imagine a shield of antioxidants guarding against oxidative stress. The Mediterranean Diet's abundance of fruits, vegetables, and olive oil provides a rich source of antioxidants, combating inflammation and reducing the risk of diabetes-related complications.

Empowering Lifestyle Choices:

8. Moderation and Mindful Eating: A Blueprint for Diabetes Care:

Envision a meal where every bite is savored, and portions are mindful. The Mediterranean Diet's emphasis on moderation and mindful eating offers a practical and enjoyable approach to managing diabetes, allowing for the pleasure of food without compromising health.

Your Journey to Balance:

As we navigate through the chapters on diabetes prevention and management in the Mediterranean Diet, consider this segment a compass, an intricate guide to a lifestyle where diabetes isn't a looming threat but a condition managed with grace and balance. Picture a life where your blood sugar levels dance in rhythm with the Mediterranean breeze, and each meal is a step towards vibrant well-being. Are you ready to embark on this journey of balance and vitality?

Cognitive Health

In the intricate landscape of well-being, cognitive health stands as the crowning jewel, an essence that defines not just our intellect but our very existence. This chapter unfolds the pages of how the Mediterranean Diet, like a nurturing gardener, tends to the flourishing garden of our minds, offering a symphony of nutrients that support mental acuity, resilience, and long-term cognitive health.

The Nutrient Symphony:

1. Omega-3 Fatty Acids: Building Blocks for Brain Vitality:

Envision a banquet where fatty fish, rich in omega-3 fatty acids, take center stage. These essential fats found abundantly in the Mediterranean Diet, serve as the foundational building blocks for brain cells, enhancing cognitive function and protecting against age-related decline.

2. Antioxidants: Shielding Against Oxidative Stress:

Picture antioxidants as guardians, shielding your brain from the oxidative stress caused by free radicals. The Mediterranean Diet, with its colorful array of fruits and vegetables, provides a robust defense against oxidative damage, supporting cognitive health.

Blood Flow and Brain Health:

3. Heart-Healthy Habits: A Boon for Brain Circulation:

Envision the heart as a conductor, orchestrating a rhythmic flow that nourishes the brain. The cardiovascular benefits of the Mediterranean Diet translate into improved blood circulation, delivering essential nutrients and oxygen to the brain, and fostering cognitive vitality.

4. Plant-Based Richness: A Bounty for Brain Health:

Picture a Mediterranean feast, rich in plant-based foods like nuts, seeds, and whole grains. These foods contribute to improved blood flow, reducing the risk of vascular damage that can compromise cognitive function.

Mindful Eating Practices:

5. Savoring Every Bite: A Mental Exercise:

Envision a meal where every bite is savored, a practice integral to the Mediterranean way of life. Mindful eating not only enhances the sensory experience but also supports cognitive function by fostering a deeper connection with the act of nourishment.

Reducing Inflammatory Crescendos:

6. Anti-Inflammatory Foods: Calming the Cognitive Symphony:

Picture inflammation as a discordant note in the cognitive symphony. The anti-inflammatory properties of the Mediterranean Diet, rooted in fruits, vegetables, and olive oil, play a crucial role in protecting the brain from chronic inflammation and associated cognitive decline.

Balancing Blood Sugar Levels:

7. Stable Blood Sugar: A Mental Equilibrium:

Envision balanced blood sugar levels as the equilibrium in your cognitive dance. The diet's emphasis on complex carbohydrates and fiber helps maintain stable blood sugar levels, reducing the risk of cognitive impairment associated with diabetes.

Your Cognitive Sonata:

As we traverse the realms of cognitive health within the Mediterranean Diet, let this chapter be a sonata, a melodic guide to nurturing the intricate orchestra of your mind. Picture a life where mental acuity and resilience are not just aspirations but tangible outcomes of a diet that cherishes the profound connection between what we eat and the vitality of our intellect. Are you ready to let the Mediterranean Diet compose a symphony of cognitive well-being in your life?

Chapter 3

Getting Started

Assessing Your Current Diet

Embarking on the journey of adopting the Mediterranean Diet is not just a change in culinary habits; it's a transformation of your relationship with food. This chapter serves as your compass, guiding you through the essential first steps, the self-reflection and assessment needed to pave the way for a sustainable and fulfilling shift toward the Mediterranean way of life.

Reflections on Your Plate:

1. Mindful Observation:

Begin this chapter with a mindful gaze at your current plate. What colors dominate? Are fruits and vegetables mere sidekicks, or do they take center stage? Reflecting on the composition of your meals lays the foundation for understanding your current dietary patterns.

2. Protein Proportions:

Assess the protein sources on your plate. Is there a balance between animal and plant-based proteins? Recognizing the protein landscape helps identify areas for adjustment and ensures you are nourishing your body with diverse sources of this essential nutrient.

Evaluating Fats:

3. Fat Content and Quality:

Delve into the fats that grace your meals. Are they predominantly saturated and trans fats, or do you incorporate heart-healthy fats like olive oil? Understanding the quality of fats in your diet is a pivotal step in aligning with the principles of the Mediterranean Diet.

The Grain Conundrum:

4. Whole Grains vs. Refined Grains:

Examine the grains that make their way to your table. Are they refined grains, stripped of their nutritional essence, or do whole grains like quinoa and brown rice take precedence? This scrutiny sets the stage for embracing the wholesome foundation of the Mediterranean Diet.

Exploring Your Relationship with Vegetables and Fruits:

5. Quantity and Variety of Plant-Based Foods:

Consider the quantity and variety of plant-based foods in your daily fare. Are fruits and vegetables abundant, offering a spectrum of nutrients, or are they overshadowed by processed options? Shifting the balance towards a plant-centric approach is a fundamental tenet of the Mediterranean Diet.

Identifying Culinary Habits:

6. Culinary Techniques and Flavor Enhancement:

Assess your culinary techniques. Are you reliant on heavy frying and excessive salt, or do you embrace the Mediterranean art of enhancing flavors with herbs, spices, and olive oil? Recognizing your cooking habits is key to making flavorful adjustments that align with the diet's principles.

Recording the Sweet Symphony:

7. Sugar Consumption:

Scrutinize your sugar consumption. Are sugary beverages and processed sweets frequent guests at your table? Acknowledging your relationship with added sugars empowers you to make conscious choices and gradually reduce your dependence on refined sweets.

Documenting Dietary Habits:
8. Keeping a Food Journal:

Consider maintaining a food journal. Documenting your daily meals and snacks provides a clear snapshot of your dietary patterns, aiding in the identification of areas that align with the Mediterranean Diet and those that may require adjustment.

Your Personalized Blueprint:

As you navigate through the process of assessing your current diet, envision this chapter as the creation of a personalized blueprint, a roadmap that not only highlights your dietary landscape but also illuminates the path toward a Mediterranean-inspired transformation. This introspective journey sets the stage for the practical steps to follow in your pursuit of optimal health and well-being. Are you ready to unfold the pages of change?

Setting Realistic Goals

In the symphony of change, setting realistic goals is the conductor that orchestrates harmony between aspiration and achievement. This chapter serves as your guide, assisting you in crafting tangible and achievable milestones on your journey toward embracing the Mediterranean Diet. Picture it as the compass that keeps you on course, ensuring your path aligns with your individual needs and aspirations.

Understanding Your Starting Point:
1. Reflection on Personal Motivations:
Begin by reflecting on why you've chosen the Mediterranean Diet. Is it for weight management, heart health, or a desire for overall well-being? Understanding your motivations lays the foundation for setting goals that resonate with your aspirations.

2. Assessing Lifestyle Constraints:
Evaluate the constraints in your current lifestyle. Are there time constraints, budget considerations, or culinary preferences that need accommodation? Identifying these factors helps in setting goals that are not only realistic but also sustainable in the long run.

Crafting S.M.A.R.T. Goals:

3. Specific Goals:

Specify your objectives. Rather than a vague goal like "eat healthier," opt for a specific target such as "consume at least five servings of vegetables daily." Clarity in your goals makes them actionable and measurable.

4. Measurable Progress:

Make your goals measurable. Quantify your objectives to track progress effectively. For instance, "reduce added sugar intake by 25% within the next month" provides a clear metric for assessment.

5. Attainable Steps:

Ensure your goals are attainable. Setting realistic targets prevents discouragement and fosters a sense of accomplishment. Instead of aiming for an extreme shift, break down your objectives into manageable steps, gradually increasing complexity as habits solidify.

6. Relevance to Your Lifestyle:

Align your goals with your lifestyle. If cooking elaborate meals is challenging, set goals that complement your routine, like "incorporate one new Mediterranean recipe into my weekly menu."

7. Time-Bound Objectives:

Set deadlines for your goals. A timeframe adds a sense of urgency and accountability. For example, "walk for 30 minutes five days a week for the next month" provides a clear time boundary.

Tailoring Goals to Your Unique Journey:

8. Personalizing Your Approach:

Recognize that everyone's journey is unique. Your goals should reflect your circumstances, health status, and preferences. A goal that suits your friend may not necessarily be the right fit for you.

9. Celebrating Milestones:

Envision your goals as a series of milestones. Celebrate achievements along the way, acknowledging the progress you've made. This positive reinforcement reinforces your commitment to the Mediterranean lifestyle.

Adapting Goals Along the Way:

10. Flexibility and Adaptability:

Acknowledge the need for flexibility. Life is dynamic, and circumstances may change. Be open to adjusting your goals as needed, ensuring they remain relevant to your evolving journey.

Your Journey, Your Rhythm:

As you navigate the process of setting realistic goals, envision this chapter as a roadmap, a compass guiding you through the terrain of change. Picture it as a flexible score, allowing for the improvisation needed to harmonize your aspirations with the realities of your unique journey. Are you ready to compose your symphony of realistic and achievable goals?

Stocking Your Mediterranean Pantry

The Mediterranean Diet is not just a collection of recipes; it's a journey woven with the threads of tradition and flavor. In this chapter, we embark on the first step of this culinary odyssey, stocking your pantry. Picture it as the canvas upon which your Mediterranean masterpiece will unfold, a treasure trove of ingredients that will infuse every meal with the sun-kissed essence of this vibrant way of life.

Foundational Staples:

1. Extra Virgin Olive Oil: The Liquid Gold:

Imagine your pantry adorned with the golden glow of extra virgin olive oil. This heart-healthy elixir is not just a cooking staple but a foundational element of the Mediterranean Diet. Opt for a high-quality, cold-pressed variety to maximize both flavor and health benefits.

2. Whole Grains: The Bedrock of Nutrition:

Picture a shelf filled with whole grains, quinoa, bulgur, farro, and brown rice. These grains form the sturdy foundation of Mediterranean meals, providing a nutrient-rich base for a variety of dishes.

3. Legumes: Protein-Packed Powerhouses:

Envision jars of beans, lentils, and chickpeas lining your shelves. Legumes are a primary protein source in the Mediterranean Diet, offering not only essential nutrients but also versatility in salads, stews, and dips.

4. Canned Tomatoes: A Burst of Sunshine:

Picture the vibrancy of canned tomatoes, sauces, diced, and crushed. These pantry heroes add depth and richness to countless Mediterranean recipes, from pasta dishes to sauces and casseroles.

Flavor Enhancers:

5. Herbs and Spices: The Mediterranean Palette:

Imagine a collection of herbs and spices transforming your dishes into flavorful masterpieces. Basil, oregano, thyme, rosemary, and garlic are the aromatic notes that define Mediterranean cuisine. Fresh or dried, they add complexity and depth to your creations.

6. Garlic and Onions: Aromatic Alchemy:

Envision baskets of garlic bulbs and bundles of onions. These aromatic ingredients form the base of many Mediterranean dishes, infusing them with rich, savory flavors.

Proteins:

7. Canned Tuna and Sardines: Seafood Staples:

Picture cans of sustainably sourced tuna and sardines. These pantry treasures are not only convenient but also provide a healthy dose of omega-3 fatty acids, supporting both cardiovascular health and cognitive function.

8. Nuts and Seeds: Nutrient-Rich Crunch:

Imagine jars filled with almonds, walnuts, and sunflower seeds. These nutrient-dense additions bring a delightful crunch to salads, yogurts, and snacks, contributing healthy fats and essential vitamins.

Condiments and Vinegar:

9. Balsamic Vinegar and Red Wine Vinegar: The Vinegar Duo:

Envision bottles of balsamic and red wine vinegar. These tangy elixirs serve as versatile dressings, marinades, and flavor enhancers, elevating the taste profile of your dishes.

10. Capers and Olives: Briny Delights:

Picture jars of capers and various types of olives, green, Kalamata, and Castelvetrano. These briny delights add a burst of flavor to salads, pasta dishes, and appetizers.

Your Mediterranean Canvas:

As you stock your Mediterranean pantry, consider this chapter a palette, a canvas upon which you'll paint the vibrant hues of your culinary exploration. Imagine the pleasure of crafting meals infused with the flavors of sun-ripened produce, aromatic herbs, and the wholesome goodness of the Mediterranean way of life. Are you ready to step into your kitchen and embark on this flavorful journey?

Chapter 4

The Mediterranean Diet Meal Plan

Breakfast Ideas

Breakfast in the Mediterranean is a celebration of simplicity and flavor, an invitation to start your day with a burst of vitality. This chapter unfolds a tapestry of breakfast ideas that not only nourish your body but also tantalize your taste buds, setting the tone for a day infused with the vibrant essence of the Mediterranean Diet.

1. Greek Yogurt Parfait with Fresh Fruit and Nuts:
Ingredients:
- Greek yogurt
- Fresh berries (strawberries, blueberries, or raspberries)
- Honey
- Chopped nuts (almonds, walnuts, or pistachios)

Preparation:

- In a glass or bowl, layer Greek yogurt with fresh berries.
- Drizzle honey over the layers for sweetness.
- Top with a generous sprinkle of chopped nuts for a delightful crunch.
- This parfait is a protein-packed, antioxidant-rich start to your day.

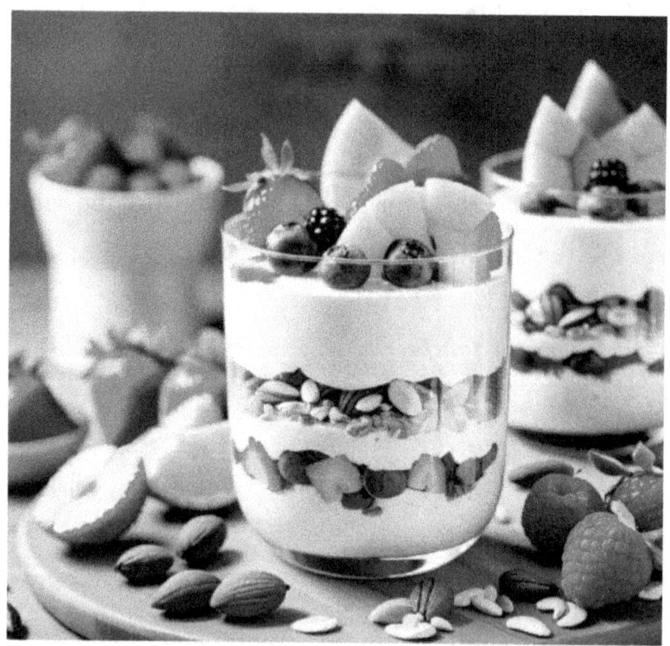

2. Avocado Toast with Tomatoes and Feta:

Ingredients:

- Whole-grain bread slices
- Ripe avocado
- Cherry tomatoes, sliced
- Feta cheese, crumbled
- Olive oil
- Fresh basil (optional)

Preparation:

- Toast whole-grain bread slices until golden.
- Mash a ripe avocado and spread it over the toast.
- Arrange sliced cherry tomatoes on top.
- Crumble feta cheese over the tomatoes.
- Drizzle with olive oil and garnish with fresh basil if desired.
- This savory toast is a nutrient-dense and satisfying option.

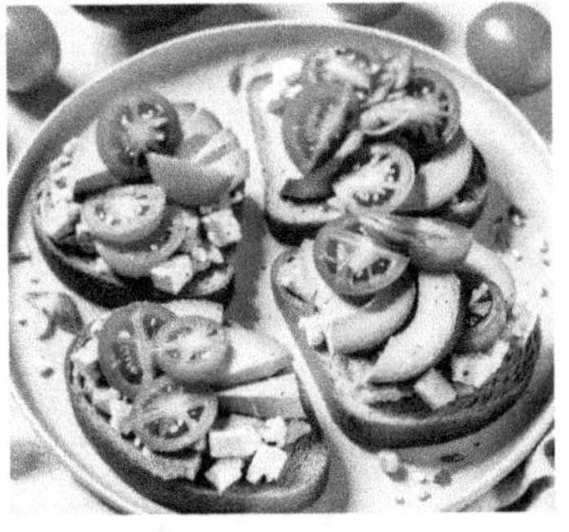

3. Mediterranean Omelette with Spinach and Feta:

Ingredients:

- Eggs
- Fresh spinach, chopped
- Feta cheese, crumbled
- Cherry tomatoes, halved
- Red onion, finely chopped
- Olive oil
- Fresh herbs (parsley or dill)

Preparation:

- In a bowl, beat eggs and season with salt and pepper.
- In a pan, sauté chopped spinach, cherry tomatoes, and red onion in olive oil until wilted.
- Pour the beaten eggs over the vegetables.
- Once the eggs set, sprinkle crumbled feta over one half and fold the omelet.
- Garnish with fresh herbs before serving.
- This protein-rich omelet is a savory and satisfying breakfast choice.

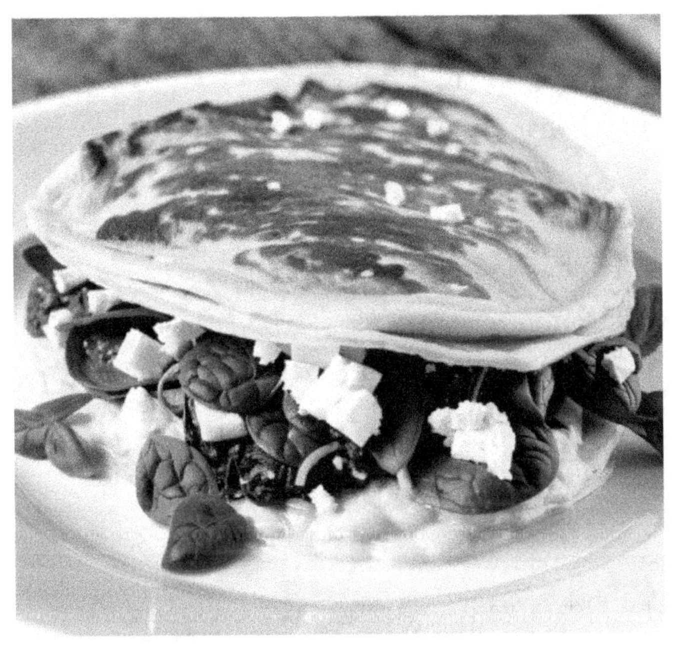

4. Whole Grain Pancakes with Fresh Berries:

Ingredients:

- Whole grain pancake mix
- Water or milk
- Fresh mixed berries
- Greek yogurt
- Honey

Preparation:

- Prepare whole grain pancakes according to the mix instructions.
- Top the pancakes with a generous dollop of Greek yogurt.
- Scatter fresh mixed berries over the yogurt.
- Drizzle with honey for sweetness.
- These pancakes offer a delightful balance of whole grains, protein, and antioxidants.

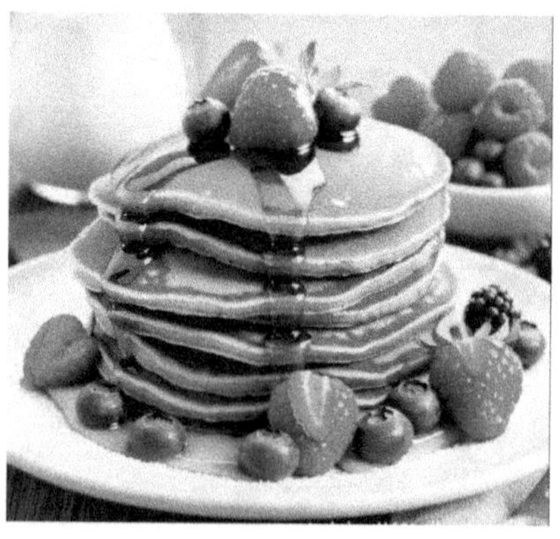

5. Chia Seed Pudding with Mango and Almonds:

Ingredients:

- Chia seeds
- Almond milk
- Mango, diced
- Sliced almonds
- Vanilla extract
- Honey

Preparation:

- Mix chia seeds with almond milk and a splash of vanilla extract.
- Let the mixture sit in the refrigerator until it thickens into a pudding-like consistency.
- Layer the chia seed pudding with diced mango.
- Top with sliced almonds and a drizzle of honey.
- This pudding is a nutrient-packed, energy-boosting breakfast.

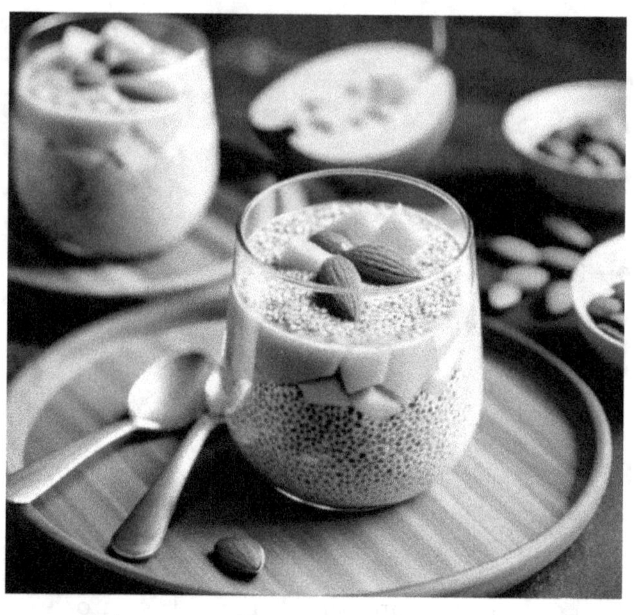

Your Breakfast Symphony:

As you dive into these Mediterranean breakfast ideas, envision this chapter as a culinary overture, a prelude to a day filled with energy, vibrancy, and the wholesome pleasure of savoring each bite. Whether you choose the refreshing parfait, the savory toast, the protein-packed omelet, the whole grain pancakes, or the nutrient-rich chia seed pudding, let breakfast be a celebration of the Mediterranean spirit. Are you ready to awaken your palate to the flavors of a Mediterranean morning?

Lunch and Dinner Recipes

Lunch and dinner in the Mediterranean are more than just meals, they are rituals, celebrations of fresh flavors, and gatherings of nourishing ingredients. This chapter unveils a repertoire of lunch and dinner recipes that not only adhere to the principles of the Mediterranean Diet but also invite you to savor the artistry of culinary harmony.

Lunch Ideas:

1. Mediterranean Chickpea Salad:
Ingredients:
- Chickpeas, cooked
- Cherry tomatoes, halved
- Cucumber, diced
- Red onion, finely chopped
- Kalamata olives, sliced
- Feta cheese, crumbled
- Fresh parsley, chopped
- Olive oil and lemon dressing

Preparation:
- Combine chickpeas, cherry tomatoes, cucumber, red onion, olives, and feta cheese in a bowl.

- Drizzle with olive oil and lemon dressing.
- Toss the ingredients gently and sprinkle with fresh parsley before serving.
- This refreshing salad is a vibrant ode to the Mediterranean palette.

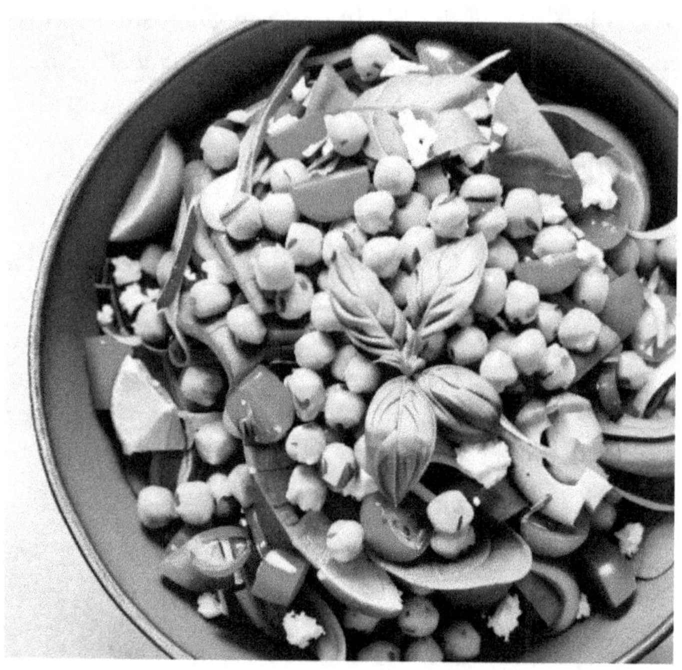

2. Grilled Mediterranean Vegetable Wrap:

Ingredients:

- Whole grain wrap
- Grilled eggplant, zucchini, and bell peppers
- Hummus
- Baby spinach leaves
- Cherry tomatoes, sliced
- Feta cheese, crumbled

Preparation:

- Spread hummus on a whole-grain wrap.
- Layer with grilled vegetables, baby spinach, cherry tomatoes, and crumbled feta.
- Roll the wrap tightly and slice it in half.
- This wrap is a delightful combination of smoky grilled veggies and Mediterranean flair.

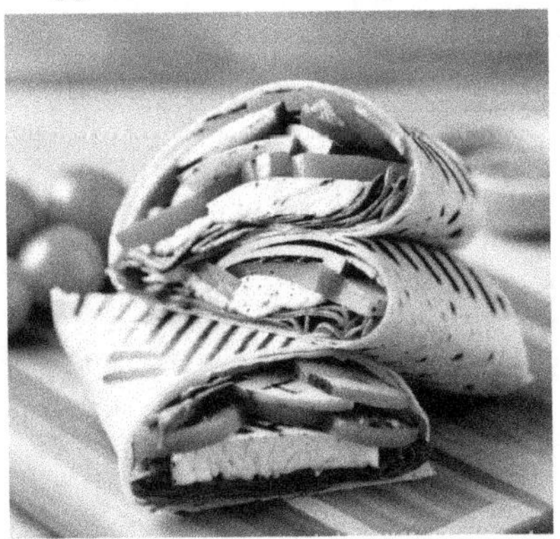

3. Lentil and Vegetable Soup:

Ingredients:

- Lentils, dried
- Carrots, diced
- Celery, chopped
- Onion, finely chopped
- Garlic, minced
- Vegetable broth
- Tomatoes, diced
- Fresh thyme and rosemary
- Olive oil

Preparation:

- Sauté onion, garlic, carrots, and celery in olive oil until softened.
- Add lentils, vegetable broth, tomatoes, and herbs.
- Simmer until lentils are tender.
- Season to taste and serve with a drizzle of olive oil.
- This hearty soup is a nourishing bowl of comfort.

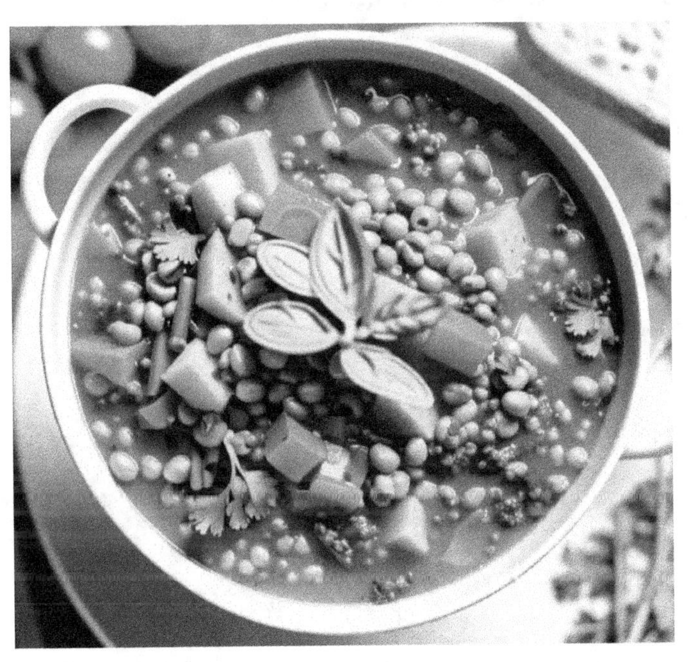

Dinner Ideas:

1. Baked Lemon Garlic Salmon:

Ingredients:

- Salmon fillets
- Lemon, sliced
- Garlic, minced
- Fresh dill, chopped
- Olive oil
- Salt and pepper

Preparation:

- Place salmon fillets on a baking sheet.
- Drizzle with olive oil and sprinkle minced garlic, fresh dill, salt, and pepper.
- Top with lemon slices.
- Bake until salmon is cooked through.
- This dish is a showcase of the Mediterranean's love affair with fresh seafood.

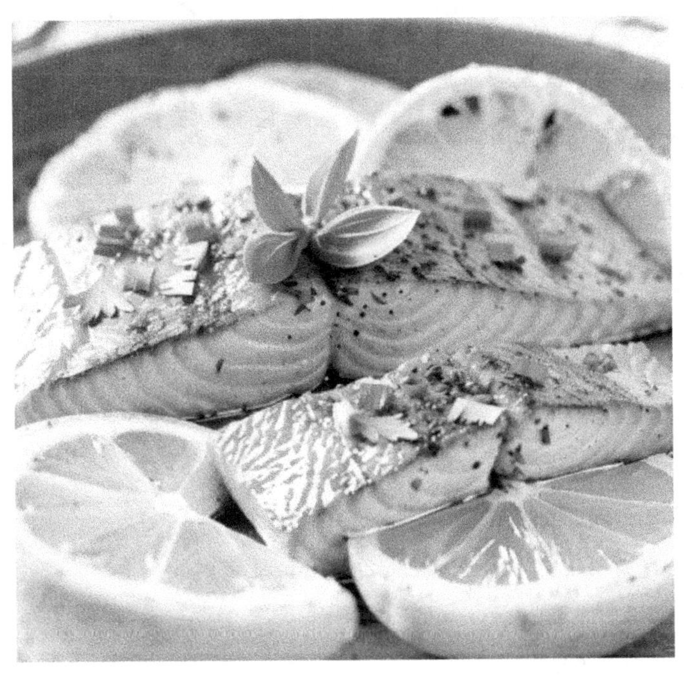

2. Quinoa and Roasted Vegetable Stuffed Peppers:
Ingredients:

- Bell peppers, halved
- Quinoa, cooked
- Roasted vegetables (zucchini, cherry tomatoes, red onion)
- Feta cheese, crumbled
- Fresh basil, chopped
- Balsamic glaze

Preparation:

- Roast vegetables until tender.
- Mix quinoa with roasted vegetables, feta, and fresh basil.
- Stuff bell peppers with the quinoa mixture.
- Bake until peppers are softened.
- Drizzle with balsamic glaze before serving.
- These stuffed peppers are a colorful and satisfying dinner option.

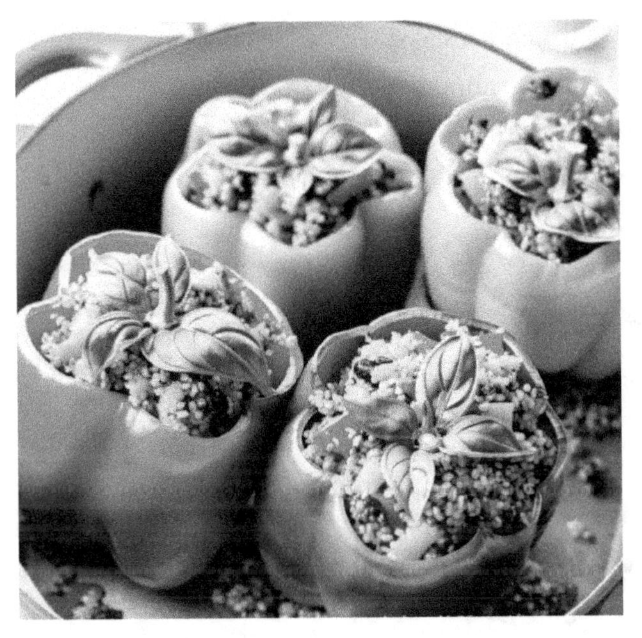

3. Eggplant and Tomato Gratin:

Ingredients:

- Eggplant, sliced
- Tomatoes, sliced
- Garlic, minced
- Fresh thyme and oregano
- Parmesan cheese, grated
- Olive oil

Preparation:

- Layer sliced eggplant and tomatoes in a baking dish.
- Sprinkle with minced garlic, fresh herbs, and Parmesan cheese.
- Drizzle with olive oil.
- Bake until the vegetables are tender and the top is golden.
- This gratin is a comforting and flavorsome Mediterranean delight.

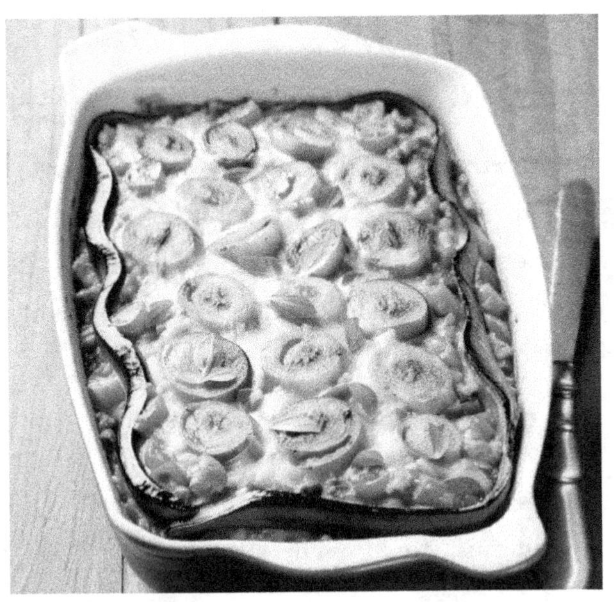

Your Culinary Odyssey:

As you explore these lunch and dinner recipes, envision this chapter as a culinary odyssey, a journey through the diverse landscapes of Mediterranean flavors. Whether you choose the vibrant chickpea salad, the grilled vegetable wrap, the comforting lentil soup, the zesty lemon garlic salmon, the quinoa-stuffed peppers, or the aromatic eggplant gratin, let each recipe be a symphony of taste that echoes the spirit of the Mediterranean way of life. Are you ready to savor the delights of a Mediterranean-inspired dinner table?

Snack Options

Snacking in the Mediterranean isn't an afterthought; it's a cherished interlude, a moment to indulge in flavors that energize and satisfy. This chapter introduces a collection of snack options that align with the principles of the Mediterranean Diet, celebrating the art of mindful nibbling and the joy of wholesome ingredients.

1. Hummus and Veggie Sticks:
Ingredients:
- Hummus (store-bought or homemade)
- Carrot sticks
- Cucumber slices
- Bell pepper strips

Preparation:
- Pair your favorite hummus with an assortment of fresh veggie sticks.
- Dip and enjoy the crispness of vegetables with the creamy goodness of hummus.
- This snack is a harmonious blend of fiber, healthy fats, and vitamins.

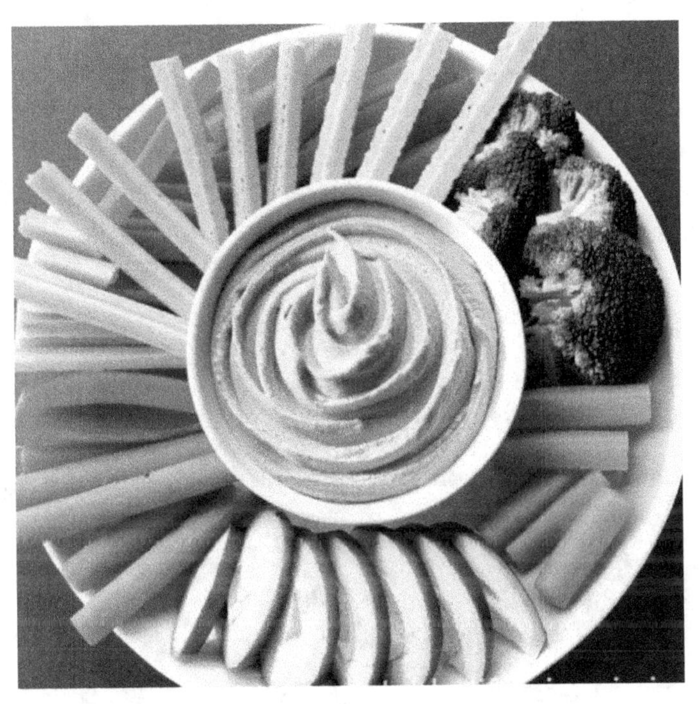

2. *Greek Yogurt with Honey and Nuts:*

Ingredients:

- Greek yogurt
- Honey
- Mixed nuts (almonds, walnuts, or pistachios)

Preparation:

- Spoon Greek yogurt into a bowl.
- Drizzle with honey for sweetness.
- Sprinkle a handful of mixed nuts for added crunch and nutrient diversity.
- This snack offers a protein-packed and satisfying combination.

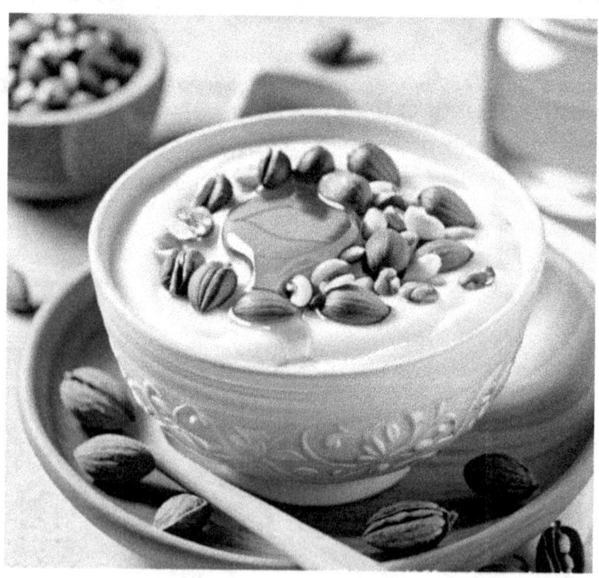

3. Roasted Chickpeas:

Ingredients:

- Canned chickpeas, drained and rinsed
- Olive oil
- Smoked paprika
- Garlic powder
- Sea salt

Preparation:

- Toss chickpeas with olive oil, smoked paprika, garlic powder, and sea salt.
- Roast in the oven until crispy.
- Allow to cool before snacking.
- These roasted chickpeas are a crunchy and fiber-rich delight.

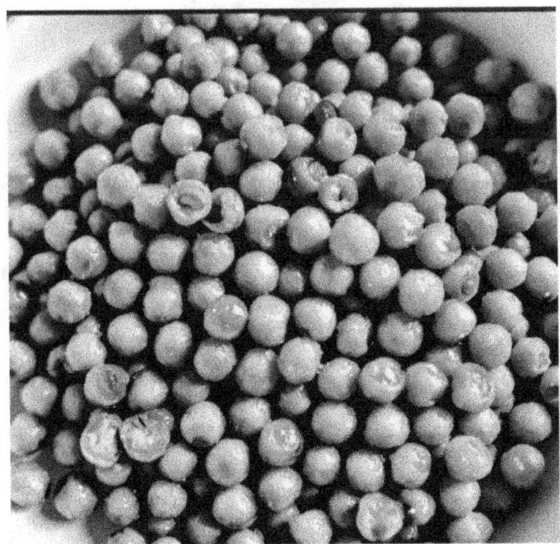

4. *Whole Grain Crackers with Feta and Tomatoes:*

Ingredients:

- Whole grain crackers
- Feta cheese, crumbled
- Cherry tomatoes, halved
- Fresh basil, chopped

Preparation:

- Arrange whole-grain crackers on a plate.
- Top each cracker with crumbled feta and a halved cherry tomato.
- Garnish with fresh basil for added flavor.
- This snack is a marriage of whole grains, calcium-rich cheese, and vibrant tomatoes.

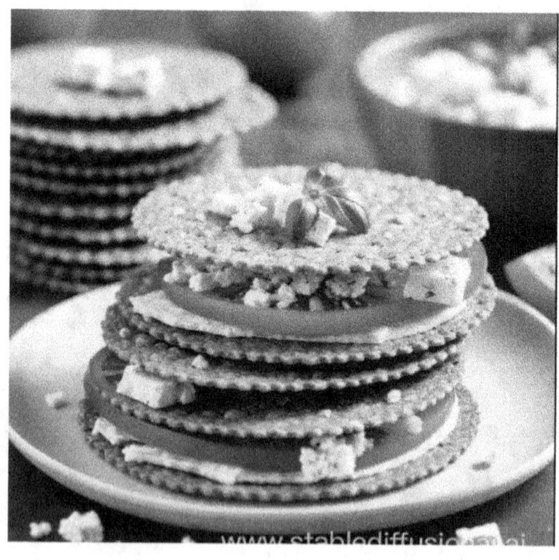

5. Mediterranean Fruit Salad:

Ingredients:

- Mixed fruits (grapes, berries, melon, citrus)
- Mint leaves, chopped
- Balsamic glaze

Preparation:

- Combine a variety of fresh fruits in a bowl.
- Sprinkle with chopped mint leaves.
- Drizzle with balsamic glaze for a sweet and tangy finish.
- This fruit salad is a refreshing and antioxidant-rich snack.

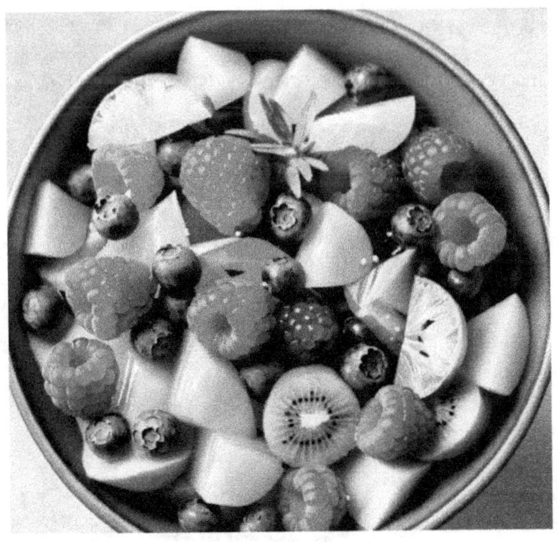

6. *Olive Tapenade with Whole Grain Toast:*

Ingredients:

- Black olives, pitted
- Kalamata olives, pitted
- Capers
- Garlic, minced
- Olive oil
- Whole grain toast

Preparation:

- Blend black olives, Kalamata olives, capers, and minced garlic in a food processor.
- Add olive oil gradually until the mixture reaches a spreadable consistency.
- Serve the olive tapenade with whole-grain toast.
- This savory spread is a delightful combination of olives and Mediterranean flavors.

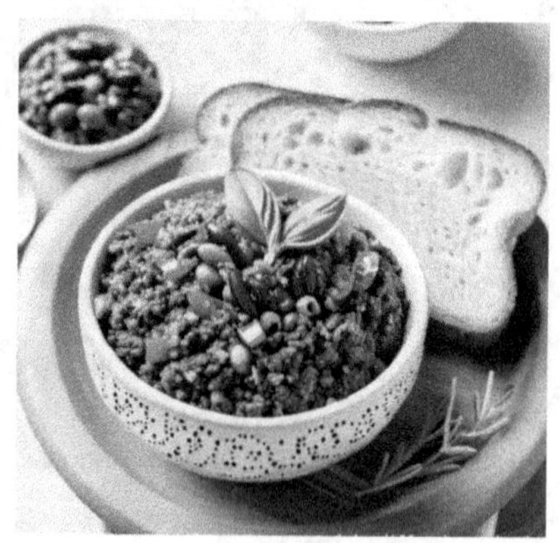

7. Dried Figs with Almonds:

Ingredients:

- Dried figs
- Almonds

Preparation:

- Pair dried figs with almonds for a sweet and nutty snack.
- This combination offers a mix of natural sugars, fiber, and healthy fats.
- Enjoy the contrasting textures and flavors in every bite.

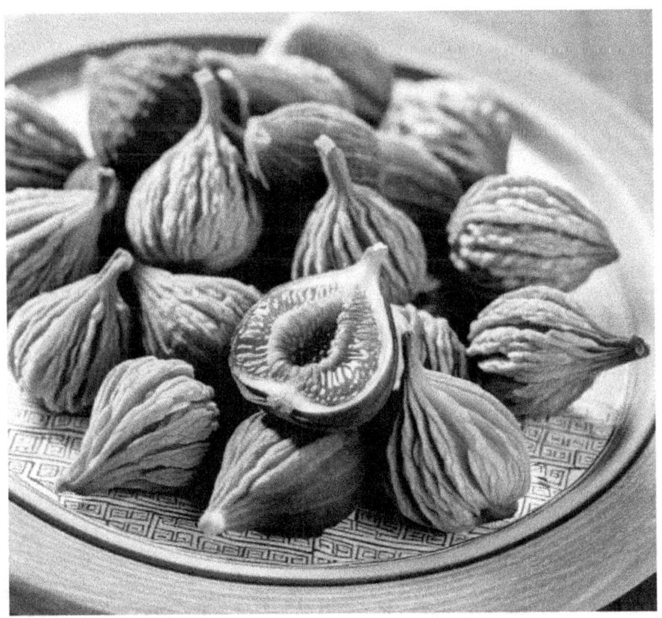

Your Snack Symphony:

As you explore these snack options, envision this chapter as a symphony, a composition of flavors that transform moments of indulgence into nourishing experiences. Whether you choose the hummus and veggie sticks, the Greek yogurt delight, the crunchy roasted chickpeas, the whole grain crackers with feta, the refreshing fruit salad, the savory olive tapenade, or the sweet pairing of dried figs and almonds, let each snack be a note in the melody of Mediterranean delights. Are you ready to savor the joy of mindful snacking?

Sample Meal Plans for Different Goals

Embarking on the Mediterranean Diet is a journey of customization, a culinary adventure where your goals become the compass guiding your food choices. This chapter presents sample meal plans tailored to different objectives, ensuring that whether you aim for weight management, cardiovascular health, or overall well-being, the Mediterranean Diet can be your compass to vibrant living.

1. Mediterranean Meal Plan for Weight Management:

Breakfast: Greek Yogurt Parfait with Fresh Berries and Almonds

Lunch:
Grilled Mediterranean Vegetable Wrap
Mixed Green Salad with Balsamic Vinaigrette

Snack: Hummus and Veggie Sticks

Dinner:
Baked Lemon Garlic Chicken Breast

Quinoa and Roasted Vegetable Stuffed Peppers
Steamed Broccoli

2. *Mediterranean Meal Plan for Cardiovascular Health:*

Breakfast: Whole Grain Pancakes with Fresh Mixed Berries

Lunch:
Mediterranean Chickpea Salad
Whole Grain Pita Bread

Snack: Greek Yogurt with Honey and Walnuts

Dinner:
Baked Salmon with Dill and Lemon
Steamed Asparagus
Brown Rice Pilaf

3. *Mediterranean Meal Plan for Overall Well-Being:*

Breakfast: Chia Seed Pudding with Mango and Almonds
Lunch:
Lentil and Vegetable Soup
Whole Grain Roll

Snack: Mediterranean Fruit Salad

Dinner:
Eggplant and Tomato Gratin
Quinoa Salad with Fresh Herbs

4. Mediterranean Meal Plan for Diabetes Management:
Breakfast: Avocado Toast with Tomatoes and Feta

Lunch:
Grilled Chicken Salad with Mixed Greens
Whole Grain Crackers with Olive Tapenade

Snack: Dried Figs with Almonds

Dinner:
Baked White Fish with Mediterranean Salsa
Sauteed Spinach with Garlic
Farro Pilaf

5. Mediterranean Meal Plan for Anti-Inflammatory Benefits:
Breakfast: Greek Yogurt Smoothie with Berries and Spinach

Lunch:

Quinoa Salad with Roasted Vegetables and Feta
Olive Oil Drizzled Whole Grain Bread

Snack: Roasted Chickpeas

Dinner:

Mediterranean Lentil Stew
Grilled Eggplant with Tahini Sauce
Wild Rice

Your Culinary Compass:

As you peruse these sample meal plans, envision this chapter as your culinary compass, a tool to navigate the diverse landscape of Mediterranean flavors while steering towards your specific health goals. Whether it's weight management, cardiovascular health, overall well-being, diabetes management, or the pursuit of anti-inflammatory benefits, let the Mediterranean Diet be your guide to a vibrant and personalized culinary journey. Are you ready to savor the tailored tastes of your Mediterranean adventure?

Chapter 5

Cooking Tips and Techniques

Flavorful Herbs and Spices

In the realm of Mediterranean cuisine, herbs and spices are the virtuosos, the alchemists that transform ordinary dishes into symphonies of flavor. This chapter delves into the artistry of using herbs and spices, offering a palette of tips and techniques that elevate your culinary creations to new heights. From the earthy notes of rosemary to the vibrant hues of saffron, let's unlock the secrets to infusing your dishes with the essence of the Mediterranean.

1. Basil: The Herb of Royalty:

Tip: Add fresh basil towards the end of cooking to preserve its delicate flavor.

Technique: Create a basil-infused olive oil by steeping fresh basil leaves in extra virgin olive oil. Drizzle this aromatic oil over salads or grilled vegetables.

2. Rosemary: The Fragrance of the Mediterranean:

Tip: Use fresh rosemary sprigs for roasting meats or vegetables.

Technique: Make rosemary skewers for kebabs by threading meat and vegetables onto sturdy rosemary branches before grilling.

3. Oregano: The Flavorful Staple:

Tip: Crush dried oregano between your fingers before adding it to release its essential oils.

Technique: Combine oregano with olive oil, garlic, and lemon juice for a quick and flavorful marinade.

4. Thyme: A Versatile Essence:

Tip: Use fresh thyme in slow-cooked dishes, allowing its flavors to meld over time.

Technique: Infuse honey with thyme by gently heating the two ingredients together. Drizzle this over desserts or incorporate it into dressings.

5. Garlic: The Aromatic Marvel:

Tip: Roast whole garlic bulbs to mellow their flavor and create a creamy consistency.

Technique: Make a garlic paste by finely mincing garlic and mixing it with a touch of salt. This paste adds depth to sauces and marinades.

6. Cilantro: Freshness Unleashed:

Tip: Chop cilantro just before using to preserve its vibrant color and flavor.

Technique: Create a cilantro pesto by blending cilantro with pine nuts, Parmesan, garlic, and olive oil. Use it as a sauce for pasta or a topping for grilled fish.

7. Saffron: The Golden Elixir:

Tip: Infuse saffron strands in warm liquid before adding to dishes for optimal color and flavor release.

Technique: Create a saffron-infused broth for paella or risotto by simmering saffron in vegetable or chicken stock.

8. Paprika: A Splash of Warmth:

Tip: Choose smoked paprika for a deeper, smokier flavor in dishes.

Technique: Dust grilled vegetables or roasted meats with paprika for a pop of color and a hint of smokiness.

9. Mint: The Refreshing Finale:

Tip: Add fresh mint to salads or desserts just before serving to maintain its brightness.

Technique: Brew a mint tea by steeping fresh mint leaves in hot water. Serve it hot or cold as a refreshing beverage.

10. Parsley: The Unsung Hero:

Tip: Use flat-leaf parsley for a more robust flavor than curly parsley.

Technique: Make a parsley gremolata by combining chopped parsley, garlic, and lemon zest. Sprinkle it over grilled meats or fish for a burst of freshness.

Your Flavorful Symphony:

As you immerse yourself in the world of flavorful herbs and spices, envision this chapter as a culinary symphony—a composition where each ingredient plays a distinct role, creating a harmonious melody of tastes and aromas. Whether it's the royal touch of basil, the fragrant allure of rosemary, or the versatile essence of oregano and thyme, let these tips and techniques be your guide to orchestrating a culinary masterpiece with the soul of the Mediterranean. Are you ready to conduct your symphony of flavors?

Healthy Cooking Oils

In the Mediterranean culinary tradition, the choice of cooking oil is as crucial as the selection of herbs and spices, a cornerstone in creating meals that are both flavorful and healthful. This chapter explores the diverse world of healthy cooking oils, guiding you through the rich array of options that bring out the best in your dishes while nourishing your body. From the golden elixir of extra virgin olive oil to the robust notes of avocado oil, let's delve into the art of choosing and using oils in the Mediterranean kitchen.

1. Extra Virgin Olive Oil: The Heartbeat of Mediterranean Cuisine:

Benefits: Rich in monounsaturated fats, antioxidants, and anti-inflammatory properties.

Cooking Use: Ideal for drizzling over salads, dipping with bread, and low to medium-heat sautéing.

2. Avocado Oil: The Green Powerhouse:

Benefits: High smoke point, heart-healthy monounsaturated fats, and a rich source of vitamins.

Cooking Use: Excellent for high-heat cooking, grilling, and roasting. Adds a subtle buttery flavor.

3. Coconut Oil: The Tropical Allure:

Benefits: High in saturated fats, including medium-chain triglycerides (MCTs), which may boost metabolism.

Cooking Use: Suitable for medium-heat cooking, baking, and frying. Adds a hint of coconut flavor.

4. Walnut Oil: The Nutty Elegance:

Benefits: Rich in omega-3 fatty acids, and antioxidants, and adds a distinctive nutty flavor.

Cooking Use: Best for drizzling over salads, vegetables, or using in dressings. Avoid high-heat cooking.

5. Sesame Oil: The Asian Infusion:

Benefits: Contains antioxidants and has a unique, nutty flavor.

Cooking Use: Use toasted sesame oil for flavoring dishes, and light sesame oil for stir-frying at medium heat.

6. Grapeseed Oil: The Light Companion:

Benefits: Mild flavor, high smoke point, and rich in polyunsaturated fats.

Cooking Use: Suitable for sautéing, frying, and as a neutral-flavored base for salad dressings.

7. Olive Oil (Light or Pure): A Versatile Alternative:

Benefits: Lighter flavor than extra virgin olive oil, suitable for various cooking methods.

Cooking Use: Can be used for sautéing, frying, and baking. A more neutral taste compared to extra virgin olive oil.

8. Flaxseed Oil: The Omega-3 Booster:

Benefits: Rich in omega-3 fatty acids, which support heart health and reduce inflammation.

Cooking Use: Best used as a finishing oil for salads or drizzling over cooked dishes. Avoid heating.

9. Canola Oil: The All-Purpose Workhorse:

Benefits: Low in saturated fat, high in smoke point, and a neutral flavor.

Cooking Use: Versatile for frying, baking, and sautéing. A common choice for its balanced profile.

10. Sunflower Oil: The Light and Neutral Option:

Benefits: High smoke point, low in saturated fats, and a neutral flavor.

Cooking Use: Suitable for frying, roasting, and baking. A versatile option for various culinary applications.

As you navigate the realm of healthy cooking oils, envision this chapter as your culinary compass, a guide to selecting the right oil for the right occasion. Whether it's the robust notes of extra virgin olive oil, the green powerhouse of avocado oil, or the tropical allure of coconut oil, let your choice of cooking oil be an intentional decision that enhances both the flavor and nutritional value of your Mediterranean-inspired creations. Are you ready to infuse your dishes with the golden elixirs of health and taste?

Cooking Methods for Maximum Nutrient Retention

In the pursuit of vibrant health, the Mediterranean way of cooking extends beyond flavor, it's about preserving the nutritional integrity of ingredients. This chapter explores cooking methods that not only bring out the rich tapestry of flavors but also ensure that the essential nutrients in your meals remain intact. From the gentle art of steaming to the quick dance of stir-frying, let's uncover the techniques that maximize the nutrient retention in every dish.

1. Steaming: The Delicate Embrace:

Method: Cooking food with steam in a covered container.

Benefits: Preserves vitamins and minerals while maintaining the natural color and texture of vegetables and seafood.

2. Grilling: The Flame-Kissed Mastery:

Method: Cooking food over an open flame or hot surface.

Benefits: Retains nutrients, enhances flavors, and imparts a smoky essence to meats, vegetables, and seafood.

3. Sautéing: The Swift Symphony:

Method: Quick cooking in a small amount of oil over medium to high heat.

Benefits: Preserves nutrient content, especially in vegetables, while developing rich flavors.

4. Roasting: The Oven's Embrace:

Method: Cooking food in an oven, usually at higher temperatures.

Benefits: Enhances natural sweetness, preserves nutrients, and creates a golden, caramelized exterior.

5. Stir-Frying: The Energetic Ballet:

Method: Rapidly cooking small, uniform-sized pieces of food in a wok or pan with oil.

Benefits: Quick cooking retains nutrients, and the minimal use of oil preserves the overall healthfulness of the dish.

6. Raw: The Pure Essence:

Method: Consuming food in its natural, uncooked state.

Benefits: Preserves enzymes, vitamins, and phytonutrients, especially in fruits, vegetables, and nuts.

7. Poaching: The Gentle Soak:

Method: Cooking food by simmering it in a liquid.

Benefits: Maintains moisture and minimizes nutrient loss, suitable for delicate proteins like fish and eggs.

8. Boiling: The Simmering Symphony:

Method: Immersing food in boiling water until cooked.

Benefits: Minimizes nutrient loss when water-soluble vitamins leach into the cooking liquid. Ideal for pasta, grains, and some vegetables.

9. Baking: The Oven's Caress:

Method: Cooking food in an oven, surrounded by dry heat.

Benefits: Suitable for dishes that benefit from longer cooking times, preserving nutrients and developing rich flavors.

10. Pressure Cooking: The Controlled Powerhouse:

Method: Using pressurized steam to cook food quickly.

Benefits: Shorter cooking times retain more nutrients, making it an efficient method for grains, legumes, and tougher cuts of meat.

Your Nutrient Symphony:

As you explore these cooking methods, envision this chapter as a nutrient symphony, a composition where each technique plays a role in preserving the vital elements of your ingredients. Whether it's the delicate embrace of steaming, the flame-kissed mastery of grilling, or the swift symphony of sautéing, let your culinary choices be a mindful dance that nourishes both body and soul. Are you ready to conduct your nutrient symphony in the Mediterranean kitchen?

Chapter 6

Navigating Challenges

Overcoming Common Obstacles

Embarking on the journey of adopting the Mediterranean lifestyle is a transformative experience, but like any adventure, it comes with its own set of challenges. This chapter serves as your guide through the common obstacles encountered on this path, offering practical insights and empowering strategies to overcome them. From time constraints to cultural adjustments, let's navigate these challenges together, ensuring a smoother voyage toward your Mediterranean-inspired lifestyle.

1. Time Constraints: The Art of Efficient Preparation:
Challenge: Busy schedules may hinder the ability to prepare elaborate Mediterranean meals.

Overcoming Strategy: Embrace batch cooking and meal prepping. Dedicate specific times during the week to prepare key components like grains, proteins, and vegetables. This ensures quick assembly of nutritious meals, even on the busiest days.

2. Access to Ingredients: Cultivating Local Connections:

Challenge: Locating authentic Mediterranean ingredients may be challenging in certain regions.

Overcoming Strategy: Explore local farmers' markets, specialty stores, or online resources to discover Mediterranean ingredients. Build connections with local suppliers and fellow enthusiasts who share a passion for the Mediterranean diet, creating a network for ingredient sourcing.

3. Cultural Shifts: Integrating Traditions with Modern Living:

Challenge: Adapting to a new culinary culture may require adjustments.

Overcoming Strategy: Gradually introduce Mediterranean flavors into your existing repertoire. Modify familiar recipes by incorporating Mediterranean ingredients and spices. Involve family members or friends in the journey, turning it into a shared cultural exploration.

4. Taste Preferences: Gradual Evolution of Palates:

Challenge: Transitioning from familiar tastes to Mediterranean flavors may pose a challenge.

Overcoming Strategy: Introduce new flavors gradually. Experiment with different herbs, spices, and ingredients, allowing your palate to adapt over time. Start with milder options and gradually incorporate bolder flavors as you become accustomed to the Mediterranean taste palette.

5. *Social Pressures: Nurturing Supportive Environments:*

Challenge: Social gatherings and events may present dietary challenges or resistance.

Overcoming Strategy: Communicate your dietary choices openly and confidently. Offer to bring a Mediterranean-inspired dish to share, ensuring there are options aligned with your preferences. Educate friends and family about the health benefits and deliciousness of the Mediterranean diet, fostering a supportive environment.

6. *Budget Constraints: Mindful Shopping and Planning:*

Challenge: The perception of Mediterranean eating as expensive may deter some individuals.

Overcoming Strategy: Plan your meals and create shopping lists to avoid impulsive purchases. Focus on seasonal, local produce and budget-friendly staples like beans, grains, and legumes. Explore cost-effective sources for olive oil and other key ingredients.

7. Culinary Skills: Embracing the Learning Curve:

Challenge: Mastering new cooking techniques and recipes can be intimidating.

Overcoming Strategy: Start with simple recipes and gradually expand your culinary skills. Utilize online resources, cookbooks, and cooking classes to enhance your knowledge. Celebrate small successes and view each cooking challenge as an opportunity for growth.

8. Sustainability Concerns: Embracing Responsible Choices:

Challenge: Balancing the desire for a Mediterranean diet with concerns about sustainability.

Overcoming Strategy: Choose sustainably sourced seafood, opt for local and seasonal produce, and support eco-friendly farming practices. Stay informed about ethical food choices and be mindful of your environmental impact while adhering to the principles of the Mediterranean diet.

Your Resilient Journey:

As you navigate through these challenges, envision this chapter as a resilient journey, a path where obstacles become stepping stones, and each challenge presents an opportunity for growth. Whether it's the art of efficient preparation, cultivating local connections, or integrating traditions into modern living, let your Mediterranean-inspired lifestyle be a dynamic and evolving adventure. Are you ready to overcome these common obstacles and embrace the transformative potential of the Mediterranean way of life?

Adapting the Diet to Dietary Restrictions

Embarking on the Mediterranean diet journey is an exciting venture, but for individuals with specific dietary restrictions, it can pose unique challenges. This chapter is your guide to navigating and adapting the Mediterranean diet to accommodate various dietary needs. Whether you follow a gluten-free, vegetarian, or lactose-free lifestyle, let's explore how the principles of the Mediterranean diet can be tailored to embrace a diverse range of dietary preferences and restrictions.

1. Gluten-Free Adaptations: Celebrating Grains and Alternatives:

Challenge: Those with gluten sensitivity or celiac disease may need to modify grain choices.

Adapting Strategy: Embrace gluten-free grains such as quinoa, brown rice, and millet. Explore alternative flours like almond flour or chickpea flour for baking. Traditional Mediterranean dishes like Greek salads, roasted vegetables, and grilled fish remain gluten-free delights.

2. Vegetarian and Vegan Transitions: Plant-Powered Abundance:

Challenge: Adapting a diet traditionally rich in seafood to a vegetarian or vegan lifestyle.

Adapting Strategy: Prioritize plant-based proteins such as beans, lentils, and tofu. Load your plate with vibrant vegetables, fruits, and whole grains. Utilize olive oil, nuts, and seeds for healthy fats. Classic Mediterranean staples like falafel, stuffed grape leaves, and vegetable-based pasta dishes can be deliciously adapted.

3. Lactose-Free Living: Embracing Dairy Alternatives:

Challenge: Navigating a diet abundant in dairy products when lactose intolerance is a concern.

Adapting Strategy: Choose lactose-free or plant-based alternatives like almond milk, coconut milk, or soy milk. Explore dairy-free versions of traditional Mediterranean dishes, such as using plant-based cheeses or yogurt alternatives. Maintain a focus on calcium-rich foods like leafy greens, fortified plant milks, and almonds.

4. Nut Allergies: Nutrient Diversity Without Nuts:

Challenge: Navigating a diet that traditionally incorporates nuts when allergies are a concern.

Adapting Strategy: Substitute seeds like sunflower seeds or pumpkin seeds for added texture and nutrients. Focus on nutrient-dense options like whole grains, legumes, and a variety of vegetables. Explore Mediterranean-inspired dishes that naturally omit nuts but still deliver a delightful array of flavors.

5. Diabetes Management: Balancing Carbohydrates and Health:

Challenge: Adapting the Mediterranean diet for individuals managing diabetes.

Adapting Strategy: Prioritize whole grains with lower glycemic indexes, such as quinoa and barley. Control portion sizes and distribute carbohydrates evenly throughout the day. Emphasize fiber-rich foods, lean proteins, and healthy fats. Mediterranean recipes can be tailored to align with diabetic dietary guidelines while retaining their delicious essence.

6. Salt Reduction: Flavorful Alternatives to Sodium:

Challenge: Reducing sodium intake, a common concern for those with hypertension or heart conditions.

Adapting Strategy: Enhance flavors with herbs, spices, and citrus to reduce reliance on salt. Choose fresh ingredients over processed options. Experiment with seasoning blends and aromatic herbs to create robust flavors without excessive sodium. The Mediterranean diet's emphasis on natural, whole foods aligns well with a lower-sodium approach.

7. Personalizing the Mediterranean Diet: Tailoring to Individual Needs:

Challenge: Addressing unique dietary restrictions or preferences beyond common categories.

Adapting Strategy: Focus on the core principles of the Mediterranean diet, whole foods, plant-based proteins, healthy fats, and a variety of colorful, seasonal ingredients. Experiment with substitutions and personalized adaptations while staying true to the spirit of the diet.

Your Adaptive Odyssey:

As you navigate the intricacies of dietary restrictions, envision this chapter as an adaptive odyssey—a journey where the Mediterranean diet becomes a canvas for personalization and creativity. Whether it's celebrating gluten-free grains, exploring plant-powered delights, embracing lactose-free alternatives, or finding flavorful alternatives to sodium, let your adaptation of the Mediterranean diet be a celebration of diversity and individuality. Are you ready to embark on your adaptive journey through the Mediterranean culinary landscape?

Chapter 7

Fitness and Lifestyle Integration

The Role of Exercise in the Mediterranean Lifestyle

The Mediterranean lifestyle isn't just about savoring delectable dishes, it's a holistic embrace of well-being, where the synergy of wholesome nutrition and regular physical activity forms the cornerstone of a vibrant life. This chapter delves into the integral role of exercise within the Mediterranean lifestyle, exploring how movement, whether through structured workouts or everyday activities, complements the diet to enhance overall health and vitality.

1. Embracing the Outdoors: Nature's Gymnasium:

Integration: The Mediterranean lifestyle celebrates the beauty of outdoor living.

Exercise Role: Engage in activities such as hiking, cycling, or swimming in the natural surroundings. This not only promotes physical fitness but also connects you with the rejuvenating energy of nature.

2. Walking: A Timeless Exercise Ritual:

Integration: Walking is a cherished and accessible daily activity.

Exercise Role: Incorporate brisk walking into your routine, whether strolling along the coastline, through vibrant markets, or amidst scenic landscapes. It's a low-impact exercise that enhances cardiovascular health.

3. Mediterranean-Inspired Workouts: Infusing Culture into Fitness:

Integration: Incorporate regional dances, such as Greek or Spanish dances, into your workout routine.

Exercise Role: These cultural workouts not only provide cardiovascular benefits but also add an element of joy and cultural richness to your fitness regimen.

4. Functional Fitness: Moving with Purpose:

Integration: The Mediterranean lifestyle emphasizes practical, purposeful movement.

Exercise Role: Include functional exercises that mimic daily activities, enhancing your strength, flexibility, and balance. This aligns with the lifestyle's emphasis on practical, everyday movement.

5. Group Activities: Community and Connection:

Integration: Social connections are vital in Mediterranean cultures.

Exercise Role: Join group activities like group hikes, yoga classes, or team sports. The camaraderie enhances motivation, making exercise a communal and enjoyable experience.

6. Water-based Activities: Fluidity and Serenity:

Integration: Proximity to the sea is a common feature in the Mediterranean.

Exercise Role: Embrace water-based activities such as swimming, kayaking, or paddleboarding. These activities not only offer a full-body workout but also provide a sense of serenity.

7. Mind-Body Practices: Harmony of Physical and Mental Wellness:

Integration: The Mediterranean lifestyle values holistic well-being.

Exercise Role: Incorporate mind-body practices like yoga or tai chi. These not only enhance flexibility and balance but also contribute to stress reduction and mental clarity.

8. Regular Movement Breaks: Elevating Daily Activities:

Integration: Infuse movement into everyday tasks.

Exercise Role: Take regular movement breaks throughout the day, whether it's stretching during work breaks, doing quick exercises at home, or opting for stairs instead of elevators. These micro-movements contribute to overall daily activity.

9. Seasonal Fitness: Harmony with Nature's Rhythms:

Integration: Seasonal changes are celebrated in Mediterranean cultures.

Exercise Role: Modify your exercise routine based on seasons. Engage in winter sports, springtime hiking, or summer swimming. This not only keeps your workouts dynamic but also aligns with the rhythm of nature.

10. Personalized Fitness Plans: Tailoring for Individual Needs:

Integration: The Mediterranean lifestyle embraces individuality.

Exercise Role: Develop a fitness plan that aligns with your preferences, fitness level, and health goals. Personalization ensures that exercise becomes a sustainable and enjoyable part of your lifestyle.

Your Active Odyssey:

As you embark on your active odyssey within the Mediterranean lifestyle, envision this chapter as a dynamic journey, a fusion of movement, culture, and well-being. Whether it's the timeless ritual of walking, the infusion of cultural workouts, or the serenity of water-based activities, let exercise become an integral part of your vibrant Mediterranean lifestyle. Are you ready to dance, walk, and flow through the enriching landscape of physical well-being?

Stress Management and Mindful Eating

In the tapestry of the Mediterranean lifestyle, stress management and mindful eating are threads that weave together to create a harmonious and healthful existence. This chapter explores the symbiotic relationship between stress, mindfulness, and the pleasures of Mediterranean cuisine, revealing how the mindful art of savoring each bite can be a powerful tool in managing stress and fostering overall well-being.

1. Understanding Stress in the Modern World:

Insight: Stress is an inevitable part of contemporary life.

Approach: Acknowledge the sources of stress, from work pressures to personal challenges, and recognize their impact on overall health.

2. Mindful Eating as a Stress-Reducing Practice:

Connection: The act of eating is deeply intertwined with stress responses.

Strategy: Embrace mindful eating, a practice that encourages present-moment awareness during meals. By savoring each bite, you can break the cycle of stress-induced eating and cultivate a healthier relationship with food.

3. *The Mediterranean Approach to Mindful Eating*:

Philosophy: Mediterranean cultures view meals as a time for connection and celebration.

Practice: Emulate the Mediterranean approach by savoring flavors, engaging in relaxed dining, and fostering a positive atmosphere during meals.

4. *Slowing Down: The Art of Paced Eating:*

Guidance: Fast-paced eating is linked to overeating and increased stress.

Practice: Adopt a slower eating pace. Take smaller bites, chew thoroughly, and allow yourself to fully experience the flavors and textures of each dish.

5. *Engaging the Senses: A Culinary Symphony:*

Awareness: Mindful eating involves engaging all the senses.

Experience: Pay attention to the colors, aromas, textures, and tastes of your food. This sensory engagement enhances the pleasure of the dining experience and promotes stress reduction.

6. *Portion Awareness: Nourishment without Excess:*

Concept: Mindful eating involves tuning into hunger and fullness cues.

Practice: Serve smaller portions, listen to your body's signals, and savor the satisfaction of being comfortably nourished without overindulgence.

7. Creating Mealtime Rituals: Moments of Tranquility:

Mindset: Mealtime rituals contribute to a sense of calm and enjoyment.

Implementation: Establish calming rituals, such as setting an inviting table, playing soft music, or expressing gratitude before meals. These practices create a serene atmosphere conducive to mindful eating.

8. Mindful Food Choices: Nourishing Body and Soul:

Discernment: Choose foods that align with both nutritional needs and personal enjoyment.

Guidance: Select a variety of fresh, seasonal, and colorful ingredients. Embrace the Mediterranean emphasis on whole foods, lean proteins, and healthy fats.

9. Stress-Reducing Nutrients: Nutritional Allies:

Awareness: Certain nutrients play a role in stress management.

Incorporation: Include foods rich in magnesium, omega-3 fatty acids, and antioxidants. These nutrients contribute to overall well-being and may have stress-reducing effects.

10. The Mindful Plate: A Reflection of Self-Care:

Shift: Transform your plate into a canvas of self-care.

Mindful Choices: With each meal, make choices that align with your health goals, personal values, and the joy of nourishing your body and soul.

Your Mindful Tapestry:

As you immerse yourself in the art of stress management and mindful eating, envision this chapter as a mindful tapestry, a weaving together of awareness, pleasure, and nourishment. Whether it's the practice of slowing down, engaging the senses, or creating mindful mealtime rituals, let each bite be a celebration of your commitment to a life filled with balance, joy, and well-being. Are you ready to savor the rich flavors of mindful living in the Mediterranean way?

*Stress management and mindful eating
are threads that weave together to create
a harmonious and healthful existence.*

Chapter 8

Anti-Aging Benefits

Nutrients for Skin Health

In the pursuit of timeless vitality, the Mediterranean lifestyle unfolds as a treasure trove of nourishment not only for the body but also for the skin. This chapter explores the anti-aging benefits embedded in the Mediterranean diet, revealing the potent nutrients that contribute to skin health. From the vibrant glow of olive oil to the antioxidant-rich embrace of colorful fruits and vegetables, let's unravel the secrets that unlock radiant, age-defying skin.

1. The Mediterranean Fountain of Youth:

Philosophy: The Mediterranean lifestyle is synonymous with graceful aging and radiant skin.

Approach: Embrace the holistic concept that beauty radiates from within, and the foods you consume play a pivotal role in nurturing the skin's health and vibrancy.

2. Olive Oil: Liquid Gold for Youthful Radiance:

Treasure: Extra virgin olive oil is a cornerstone of the Mediterranean diet.

Benefits: Rich in monounsaturated fats and antioxidants, olive oil nourishes the skin, maintains elasticity, and provides a natural glow. Incorporate it into cooking and drizzle it over salads for a daily dose of skin-loving goodness.

3. Omega-3 Fatty Acids: The Elixir of Youth:

Essentials: Fatty fish, walnuts, and flaxseeds are omega-3-rich sources.

Benefits: Omega-3 fatty acids support skin elasticity, and hydration, and may alleviate inflammation. Include fatty fish like salmon, mackerel, and sardines in your diet for a powerful anti-aging boost.

4. Colorful Fruits and Vegetables: Nature's Anti-Aging Palette:

Vibrance: The Mediterranean diet celebrates the rainbow of produce.

Benefits: High in vitamins, minerals, and antioxidants, colorful fruits and vegetables combat oxidative stress, reducing the signs of aging. Incorporate tomatoes, berries, leafy greens, and peppers for a vibrant skin-enhancing spectrum.

5. Nuts and Seeds: Nutrient-Rich Beauty Bites:

Treasures: Almonds, sunflower seeds, and pumpkin seeds are nutrient-dense options.

Benefits: Packed with vitamin E, zinc, and antioxidants, nuts and seeds support skin health by combating oxidative damage. Snack on a handful or sprinkle them over salads and yogurt for an anti-aging crunch.

6. Lean Proteins: Building Blocks of Youthful Skin:

Sources: Include lean proteins such as poultry, legumes, and tofu.

Benefits: Amino acids from lean proteins contribute to collagen synthesis, promoting skin elasticity and firmness. Opt for a variety of protein sources for a well-rounded approach to anti-aging.

7. Hydration from Within: The Elixir of Youth:

Nectar: Water is the ultimate hydrating elixir.

Benefits: Adequate hydration is essential for plump, supple skin. In the Mediterranean tradition, water is a fundamental component of daily living. Sip water throughout the day to maintain skin hydration and vitality.

8. Red Wine: A Toast to Skin Health:

Elixir: Red wine, consumed in moderation, is a symbol of Mediterranean conviviality.

Benefits: Rich in antioxidants, particularly resveratrol, red wine may contribute to improved skin elasticity and protection against environmental stressors. Enjoy a glass occasionally as part of a balanced lifestyle.

9. Green Tea: Sip to Rejuvenate:

Infusion: Green tea is a staple in Mediterranean regions.

Benefits: Abundant in polyphenols and catechins, green tea exhibits anti-inflammatory and antioxidant properties, contributing to skin health. Incorporate this soothing elixir into your daily routine.

10. Dark Chocolate: Indulgence with Benefits:

Treat: Dark chocolate, in moderation, can be a delightful addition.

Benefits: Packed with flavonoids, dark chocolate may enhance skin hydration and protect against sun damage. Opt for high-quality, minimally processed dark chocolate for a guilt-free treat.

Your Age-Defying Feast:

As you savor the nutrients for skin health embedded in the Mediterranean diet, envision this chapter as an age-defying feast, a banquet of flavors that not only tantalize your taste buds but also nourish and rejuvenate your skin from within. Whether it's the liquid gold of olive oil, the omega-3 elixir from fatty fish, or the vibrant hues of fruits and vegetables, let each bite be a step toward timeless radiance. Are you ready to indulge in the beauty-enhancing bounty of the Mediterranean diet?

Longevity and the Mediterranean Diet

In the heartlands of the Mediterranean, where time seems to slow and traditions endure, a powerful connection between the diet and longevity unfolds. This chapter delves into the fascinating interplay between the Mediterranean diet and the pursuit of a long, vibrant life. From the wisdom of centenarian communities to the nourishing embrace of olive groves, let's explore the secrets that unlock the door to a life well-lived.

1. Centenarian Wisdom: Learning from the Elders:

Inspiration: Mediterranean regions boast a high number of centenarians.

Insight: Explore the habits and dietary patterns of these long-lived individuals, drawing inspiration from their simple yet profound approach to life.

2. Plant-Centric Brilliance: The Green Foundation:

Cornerstone: Plant-based foods form the essence of the Mediterranean diet.

Impact: High consumption of fruits, vegetables, legumes, and whole grains provides essential nutrients and antioxidants, contributing to overall health and longevity.

3. Olive Oil: Liquid Gold of Longevity:

Treasure: Extra virgin olive oil is a staple in Mediterranean kitchens.

Power: Rich in monounsaturated fats and antioxidants, olive oil supports heart health, reduces inflammation, and may contribute to longevity. Make it a daily companion in your culinary journey.

4. Seafood Sustenance: Omega-3 Rich Oceans:

Bounty: Fatty fish like salmon, sardines, and mackerel are Mediterranean delicacies.

Benefit: Omega-3 fatty acids from seafood promote cardiovascular health, reduce inflammation, and are associated with increased longevity. Include fish in your diet regularly for a maritime boost.

5. Modest Portions: Savoring the Essence:

Practice: The Mediterranean approach emphasizes moderation in portion sizes.

Impact: Consuming smaller, balanced portions may contribute to maintaining a healthy weight, reducing the risk of chronic diseases, and supporting longevity.

6. Rituals of Communal Dining: Social Nourishment:

Tradition: Shared meals are central to Mediterranean culture.

Effect: Communal dining fosters strong social bonds, reducing feelings of isolation and promoting mental well-being, an essential aspect of a long, fulfilling life.

7. Red Wine in Moderation: A Toast to Health:

Cultural Symbol: Red wine is a symbol of conviviality in the Mediterranean.

Benefit: Moderate consumption of red wine, rich in antioxidants like resveratrol, is associated with heart health and longevity. Savor a glass with meals as part of a balanced lifestyle.

8. Herbal Infusions: Nature's Elixirs:

Cultural Practice: Herbal teas, like chamomile and mint, are prevalent in Mediterranean cultures.

Contribution: Herbal infusions offer a range of health benefits, from digestion to relaxation, contributing to overall well-being and longevity.

9. Active Living: Nature's Gymnasium:

Lifestyle Choice: Regular physical activity is integrated into daily life.

Impact: Engaging in activities like walking, gardening, and outdoor pursuits not only enhances physical health but also contributes to mental and emotional well-being, fostering longevity.

10. Stress Management: Serenity for the Soul:

Philosophy: The Mediterranean lifestyle values a balanced, relaxed approach to life.

Practice: Implement stress-reducing practices, such as mindfulness, yoga, or moments of tranquility, to promote emotional health, a key element in the pursuit of a long, fulfilling life.

Your Symphony of Longevity:

As you immerse yourself in the symphony of longevity embedded in the Mediterranean diet, envision this chapter as a harmonic journey, a composition of flavors, traditions, and lifestyle choices that harmonize to create a life of enduring vitality. Whether it's the wisdom of centenarians, the green brilliance of plant-centric meals, or the communal joy of shared dining, let each note resonate as you conduct your symphony of longevity. Are you ready to dance through the pages of a life well-lived in the Mediterranean tradition?

Chapter 9

Maintaining Progress

Staying Motivated

Embarking on the journey toward optimal health, weight loss, and well-being is a transformative experience, but the real challenge lies in sustaining the progress achieved. This chapter delves into the art of maintaining your newfound lifestyle, offering insights and strategies to keep your motivation high. From cultivating positive habits to navigating setbacks, let's explore the keys to longevity in your journcy to a healthier and more vibrant you.

1. The Momentum of Habits: Cultivating Positive Routines:

Insight: Sustainable progress often hinges on the power of habits.

Strategy: Identify and nurture positive habits developed on your journey. From mindful eating to regular exercise, let these habits become the backbone of your ongoing success.

2. Goal Reassessment: Celebrating Milestones, Setting New Targets:

Reflection: Celebrate the achievements that mark your progress.

Action: Periodically reassess your goals, acknowledging milestones and setting new targets. This dynamic approach keeps your journey fresh and engaging.

3. Accountability Partners: Sharing the Journey:

Community: Share your goals and progress with a supportive network.

Support: Accountability partners, whether friends, family, or fellow enthusiasts, provide encouragement and motivation. Discuss challenges, celebrate successes, and reinforce your commitment together.

4. Diversifying Your Routine: Embracing Variety:

Engagement: Monotony can lead to boredom and decreased motivation.

Adaptation: Regularly introduce variety into your routine. Explore new recipes, try different forms of exercise, or engage in diverse activities to keep your journey dynamic and enjoyable.

5. *Mindful Indulgences: Balancing Pleasure and Progress:*

Philosophy: Allow room for occasional indulgences without guilt.

Balance: Incorporate treats mindfully, savoring them as part of a balanced lifestyle. This approach fosters a positive relationship with food and promotes long-term adherence to your health goals.

6. *Regular Progress Assessments: Tracking Your Journey:*

Awareness: Regularly assess your progress and adjust as needed.

Adjustment: Monitoring your achievements and challenges allows you to fine-tune your approach. Keep a journal, take measurements, or use apps to track your journey over time.

7. *Continued Education: Nourishing Your Knowledge:*

Curiosity: Cultivate a curious mindset about nutrition, fitness, and well-being.

Learning: Stay informed about the latest research, recipes, and wellness practices. This ongoing education not only reinforces your commitment but also keeps your journey exciting and evolving.

8. Flexibility in Approach: Adapting to Life's Flux:

Realism: Life is dynamic, and adaptability is key to maintaining progress.

Mindset: Embrace a flexible approach to your lifestyle. Allow for adjustments during busy periods or unforeseen challenges, ensuring that your journey remains sustainable in the long run.

9. Reflecting on Non-Scale Victories: Beyond the Numbers:

Appreciation: Acknowledge and celebrate non-scale victories.

Perspective: Shift your focus beyond weight alone. Recognize improvements in energy levels, mood, sleep quality, and overall well-being, fostering a holistic perspective on your journey.

10. Resilience in Setbacks: Learning from Challenges:

Reality: Setbacks are a natural part of any journey.

Mindset: Approach setbacks as learning opportunities. Analyze what led to the setback, adapt your strategy, and use the experience to reinforce your resilience and commitment.

Your Ever-Evolving Journey:

As you navigate the terrain of maintaining progress, envision this chapter as a compass guiding your ever-evolving journey, a compass that directs you through the highs and lows with resilience and determination. Whether it's cultivating positive habits, reassessing goals, or celebrating non-scale victories, let each step be a testament to your commitment to lasting well-being. Are you ready to continue dancing along the path of sustained progress and vibrant living?

Fine-Tuning Your Approach

In the symphony of a health and well-being journey, fine-tuning your approach becomes the conductor's baton, shaping the nuances that define your experience. This chapter delves into the art of refining and optimizing your strategy, offering insights and practical tips to enhance the effectiveness and sustainability of your chosen path. From nutritional adjustments to personalized fitness tweaks, let's explore the delicate balance of fine-tuning for a harmonious and vibrant lifestyle.

1. Reflecting on Personal Preferences: Tailoring for Enjoyment:

Exploration: Revisit your chosen dietary and fitness elements.

Adjustment: Fine-tune your approach by aligning it with your personal preferences. Choose foods and activities you genuinely enjoy, ensuring that your journey remains fulfilling and sustainable.

2. Nutritional Adjustments: Adapting to Your Body's Signals:

Awareness: Listen to your body's responses to your current nutritional plan.

Refinement: Fine-tune your diet based on how your body reacts to certain foods. Adjust portion sizes, nutrient ratios, or meal timing to optimize energy levels and overall well-being.

3. Customizing Your Fitness Routine: Personalizing Movement:

Assessment: Evaluate the effectiveness and enjoyment of your current exercise regimen.

Modification: Fine-tune your fitness routine by incorporating activities that resonate with your preferences. This may involve trying new workouts, adjusting intensity, or exploring different forms of movement.

4. Sleep Optimization: Enhancing Rest and Recovery:

Importance: Quality sleep is integral to overall health.

Adjustment: Fine-tune your sleep routine by creating a conducive environment, establishing a consistent sleep schedule, and minimizing screen time before bedtime. Adequate rest supports physical and mental well-being.

5. Stress Management Strategies: Refining Relaxation Techniques:

Stress Awareness: Identify sources of stress in your life.

Technique Refinement: Fine-tune your stress management techniques. Experiment with mindfulness, deep breathing, or other relaxation methods to discover what resonates most effectively with you.

6. *Hydration Optimization: Nurturing Fluid Balance:*

Hydration Awareness: Pay attention to your daily fluid intake.

Fine-tuning: Adjust your hydration strategy based on factors such as climate, activity level, and individual needs. Optimal hydration supports various bodily functions and contributes to overall well-being.

7. *Mindful Eating Practices: Elevating Culinary Awareness:*

Present-Moment Awareness: Revisit the practice of mindful eating.

Refinement: Fine-tune your approach by incorporating mindful eating techniques. Chew slowly, savor each bite, and pay attention to hunger and fullness cues. This fosters a deeper connection with your meals.

8. *Goal Realignment: Aligning Aspirations with Reality:*

Goal Reflection: Assess the alignment of your goals with your current lifestyle.

Adjustment: Fine-tune your goals to ensure they are realistic and achievable. Setting objectives that resonate with your present circumstances enhances motivation and success.

9. *Social Support Enhancement: Strengthening Connections:*

Community Check: Reevaluate your support network.

Connection Cultivation: Fine-tune your social support system by actively engaging with friends, family, or like-minded individuals who share your health and well-being goals. A supportive community enhances motivation and accountability.

10. *Consistency Calibration: Balancing Routines:*

Routine Analysis: Examine the consistency of your health routines.

Calibration: Fine-tune your approach by balancing consistency with flexibility. While regularity is crucial, allows room for adaptability to prevent monotony and enhance sustainability.

Your Symphony of Wellness:

As you navigate the delicate process of fine-tuning your approach, envision this chapter as a conductor's score—a dynamic arrangement of choices, adjustments, and harmonies that compose your symphony of wellness. Whether it's reflecting on personal preferences, refining stress management, or optimizing sleep, let each refined note contribute to the melodic journey of a vibrant and balanced life. Are you ready to step into the spotlight and conduct the ongoing masterpiece of your well-being?

Seeking Professional Guidance

In the tapestry of wellness, seeking professional guidance emerges as a compass, guiding you through the complexities of your health journey. This chapter explores the invaluable role of experts in nutrition, fitness, and mental well-being, shedding light on how their guidance can enhance your understanding, motivation, and overall success. From registered dietitians to fitness trainers, and mental health professionals to healthcare providers, let's delve into the collaborative dance between seekers and guides in the pursuit of optimal health.

1. The Expert's Palette: Understanding Professional Roles:

Clarity: Discern the distinct roles of various health professionals.

Insight: Gain an understanding of how registered dietitians, fitness trainers, mental health professionals, and healthcare providers contribute to different facets of your well-being.

2. Nutritional Guidance: The Role of Registered Dietitians:

Expertise: Registered dietitians are trained nutrition experts.

Consultation: Seek a registered dietitian for personalized nutritional guidance. They can assess your dietary needs, offer tailored recommendations, and provide ongoing support for achieving your health goals.

3. Fitness Training Expertise: Collaborating with Trainers:

Proficiency: Fitness trainers bring expertise in exercise programming.

Partnership: Engage with a fitness trainer to design a customized workout plan aligned with your goals. Their guidance ensures proper form, progression, and motivation in your fitness journey.

4. Mental Health Professionals: Nurturing Emotional Well-Being:

Specialization: Psychologists, counselors, and therapists specialize in mental health.

Support: Consider consulting mental health professionals for emotional well-being. They provide strategies for stress management, coping with challenges, and fostering a positive mindset.

5. Healthcare Providers: The Pillars of Physical Health:

Comprehensive Care: Physicians, nurses, and healthcare providers offer holistic health perspectives.

Check-ins: Schedule regular check-ups with healthcare providers to monitor physical health, discuss preventive measures, and address any medical concerns. Their insights contribute to a well-rounded approach to wellness.

6. Holistic Approaches: Integrative and Functional Medicine:

Approach: Integrative and functional medicine practitioners explore holistic well-being.

Consultation: Consider integrative or functional medicine professionals for a comprehensive approach that considers lifestyle, nutrition, and individual health factors.

7. Wellness Coaches: Guiding the Journey:

Guidance: Wellness coaches provide support in various areas of well-being.

Partnership: Engage with a wellness coach for motivation, goal setting, and accountability. Their holistic approach can align with your broader vision for a healthy lifestyle.

8. Collaborative Care: The Interconnected Web of Health Professionals:

Communication: Foster collaboration between different health professionals.

Integration: Ensure that professionals across various domains communicate to create a cohesive, integrated plan. This collaborative approach addresses your unique health needs more comprehensively.

9. *Assessing Credentials: Navigating the Expert Landscape:*

Evaluation: Scrutinize the credentials and qualifications of health professionals.

Research: Ensure that the professionals you consult hold recognized certifications and qualifications in their respective fields. This due diligence ensures that you receive reliable and evidence-based guidance.

10. *Ongoing Education: Empowering Yourself through Knowledge:*

Empowerment: Take an active role in your health journey by staying informed.

Learning: Continuously educate yourself about nutrition, fitness, and mental health. This knowledge empowers you to actively engage in discussions with health professionals and make informed decisions about your well-being.

Chapter 10

Recipes from the Mediterranean

Classic Dishes

Embarking on a culinary journey through the Mediterranean is like setting sail on a flavorful odyssey where each dish narrates a tale of tradition, taste, and timeless joy. This chapter invites you into the heart of Mediterranean kitchens, presenting classic recipes that capture the essence of this renowned cuisine. From the aromatic herbs of Greece to the sun-soaked tomatoes of Italy, let's explore the artistry of preparing iconic dishes that bring the Mediterranean lifestyle to your table.

1. Greek Moussaka: Layers of Mediterranean Delight

Inspiration: Inspired by the layers of Greek culture and flavors.

Ingredients: Eggplant, minced meat, tomatoes, béchamel sauce.

Preparation: Sliced eggplant is layered with a savory meat sauce, topped with a creamy béchamel, and baked to golden perfection. A taste of Greece in every bite.

2. *Italian Pasta Puttanesca: A Symphony of Mediterranean Flavors*

Inspiration: Evoking the vibrant spirit of Italian coastal cuisine.

Ingredients: Tomatoes, olives, capers, garlic, anchovies.

Preparation: This boldly flavored pasta dish is a harmonious blend of tomatoes, olives, capers, and anchovies. A quick and savory symphony that transports you to the sun-soaked shores of Italy.

3. *Spanish Paella: Saffron-Kissed Sensation*

Inspiration: Drawing from the rich culinary tapestry of Spain.

Ingredients: Rice, saffron, chicken, seafood, vegetables.

Preparation: A fragrant rice dish simmered with saffron and an array of proteins like chicken, rabbit, and seafood. Paella captures the essence of Spanish coastal living in a single, flavorful pan.

4. *Provencal Ratatouille: Colorful Harmony of Vegetables*

Inspiration: Infused with the rustic charm of Provence, France.

Ingredients: Eggplant, zucchini, bell peppers, tomatoes, herbs.

Preparation: A vegetable medley cooked to perfection, Ratatouille embodies the simplicity and bounty of the French countryside. Layers of vibrant vegetables meld together in a celebration of Provencal flavors.

5. *Turkish Kebabs: Grilled Perfection*

Inspiration: Reflecting the vibrant street food culture of Turkey.

Ingredients: Marinated meats (beef, lamb, or chicken), spices.

Preparation: Marinated and skewered meats, grilled to smoky perfection. Whether adana, shish, or döner, Turkish kebabs showcase the art of grilling and the bold flavors of Turkish cuisine.

6. *Moroccan Tagine: Slow-Cooked Elegance*

Inspiration: Echoing the slow-cooked traditions of Morocco.

Ingredients: Meat (lamb, chicken), vegetables, dried fruits, spices.

Preparation: A stew-like dish cooked in a distinctive earthenware pot, a tagine blends savory meats, aromatic spices, and sweet dried fruits. A rich and comforting taste of Morocco.

7. Lebanese Tabbouleh: Freshness in Every Bite

Inspiration: Drawing from the vibrant mezze culture of Lebanon.

Ingredients: Bulgar wheat, parsley, tomatoes, mint, lemon.

Preparation: A refreshing salad bursting with herbs, Tabbouleh is a zesty concoction of bulgur wheat, fresh vegetables, and a citrusy dressing. A Lebanese classic that adds a crisp, palate-cleansing note to any meal.

8. Sicilian Cannoli: Sweet Sicilian Indulgence

Inspiration: Reflecting the sweet traditions of Sicily.

Ingredients: Ricotta, sugar, pistachios, chocolate.

Preparation: Crispy pastry tubes filled with sweetened ricotta and adorned with pistachios or chocolate. Sicilian Cannoli epitomizes the irresistible allure of Mediterranean desserts.

9. Croatian Pasticada: Slow-Simmered Elegance

Inspiration: A Croatian dish that captures the essence of coastal living.

Ingredients: Beef, prunes, vegetables, red wine.

Preparation: A slow-cooked beef stew, Pasticada blends savory meats with the sweetness of prunes and the depth of red wine. A dish that reflects the culinary finesse of Croatia.

10. Israeli Hummus: Creamy Middle Eastern Delight

Inspiration: Rooted in the Middle Eastern culinary heritage.

Ingredients: Chickpeas, tahini, garlic, lemon.

Preparation: A velvety blend of chickpeas, tahini, garlic, and lemon, Hummus is a Middle Eastern staple that epitomizes simplicity and taste. Spread it on a warm pita or serve as a flavorful dip.

Your Mediterranean Feast:

As you embark on the culinary odyssey of preparing these classic Mediterranean dishes, envision this chapter as a feast, an abundant table laden with the diverse flavors, textures, and stories that define the rich tapestry of Mediterranean cuisine. Whether you're savoring the layers of Moussaka, the grilled perfection of Turkish Kebabs, or the creamy delight of Israeli Hummus.

Modern Variations

In the ever-evolving landscape of culinary artistry, the Mediterranean classics serve as a canvas for innovation and contemporary flair. This chapter invites you to explore modern variations on traditional favorites, where creative twists and fresh perspectives breathe new life into timeless recipes. From inventive ingredient pairings to innovative cooking techniques, let's embark on a gastronomic journey that pays homage to tradition while embracing the excitement of the culinary present.

1. Deconstructed Greek Salad: A Visual Symphony

Inspiration: Drawing from the vibrant colors of a Greek salad.

Variation: Deconstruct the classic Greek salad, arranging tomatoes, cucumbers, olives, and feta in an artful display. Drizzle with a balsamic reduction for a visually stunning and flavor-packed twist.

2. Lemon Infused Pasta Puttanesca: A Citrusy Twist

Inspiration: Evoking the bold flavors of Italian Puttanesca.

Variation: Infuse the traditional pasta Puttanesca with a burst of citrus by adding fresh lemon zest. The lemony brightness enhances the robust flavors of olives, capers, and anchovies.

3. Quinoa Paella with Chorizo: A Grainy Rendition

Inspiration: Paying homage to the Spanish classic, Paella.

Variation: Replace traditional rice with nutrient-rich quinoa and add flavorful chorizo for a protein-packed twist on the beloved Spanish dish. A modern paella that combines tradition with nutritional innovation.

4. Roasted Vegetable Ratatouille Tart: Puff Pastry Elegance

Inspiration: Inspired by the layered beauty of Provencal Ratatouille.

Variation: Transform Ratatouille into an elegant tart by arranging roasted vegetables atop a delicate puff pastry. Each slice unveils a colorful mosaic of flavors and textures.

5. Grilled Halloumi Kebabs: Mediterranean Fusion

Inspiration: Building on the grilled perfection of Turkish Kebabs.

Variation: Swap traditional meats with halloumi cheese, threading it onto skewers alongside vibrant vegetables. Grilled to perfection, these halloumi kebabs offer a delightful vegetarian twist.

6. *Moroccan-Inspired Quinoa Tagine: A Grainful Melange*

Inspiration: Infusing the essence of Morocco into a quinoa-based tagine.

Variation: Replace traditional grains with quinoa in a Moroccan tagine, marrying the aromatic spices with the nutty goodness of quinoa. A modern, protein-packed interpretation.

7. *Kale Tabbouleh: A Leafy Resurgence*

Inspiration: Reimagining the freshness of Lebanese Tabbouleh.

Variation: Introduce nutrient-rich kale into Tabbouleh for a leafy and vibrant variation. The robust flavors of kale complement the traditional herbs, creating a modern twist on this classic salad.

8. *Cannoli Dip with Berries: Dessert Unplugged*

Inspiration: Embracing the sweet indulgence of Sicilian Cannoli.

Variation: Transform the beloved Sicilian Cannoli into a delightful dip. Serve with fresh berries for a light and shareable dessert that captures the essence of the original.

9. Modern Pasticada Sliders: Bite-Sized Elegance

Inspiration: Drawing from the slow-cooked elegance of Croatian Pasticada.

Variation: Transform Pasticada into bite-sized sliders, featuring tender beef, prunes, and a savory reduction between miniature buns. A modern, elegant twist on a traditional Croatian dish.

10. Roasted Red Pepper Hummus: A Vibrant Spin

Inspiration: Building on the creamy delight of Israeli Hummus.

Variation: Infuse traditional hummus with the smoky sweetness of roasted red peppers. This vibrant spin adds depth and a pop of color to the classic Middle Eastern dip.

Your Culinary Canvas:

As you explore these modern variations on Mediterranean classics, envision this chapter as a culinary canvas, a space where tradition meets innovation, and each dish is a brushstroke of contemporary flair. Whether savoring the visual symphony of a deconstructed Greek salad or the bite-sized elegance of modern Pasticada sliders, let each dish be a testament to the evolving tapestry of Mediterranean cuisine. Bon appétit!

Conclusion

As we reach the final pages of "The Mediterranean Diet Decoded: Your Comprehensive Guide to Achieving Optimal Health, Weight Loss, and Anti-Aging Benefits," we've embarked on a rich and flavorful odyssey through the heartlands of Mediterranean living. From the sun-drenched shores of Greece to the rustic kitchens of Provence, each chapter has unfolded a tapestry of traditions, flavors, and well-being practices.

In decoding the principles of the Mediterranean diet, understanding its science-backed effectiveness, and exploring the diverse health benefits, you've gained insights into a lifestyle that extends beyond the plate. This journey has not merely been about food; it's been a celebration of a holistic approach to health, one that embraces physical well-being, mental vitality, and the joy of communal living.

As we delved into the practical aspects of getting started, setting realistic goals, and navigating the challenges inherent in any wellness journey, you've equipped yourself with tools that go beyond mere knowledge. They are the building blocks of lasting habits, resilience, and a positive mindset, the pillars that sustain progress.

Your exploration of classic Mediterranean recipes, both traditional and modern, has transformed your kitchen into a canvas, where each dish tells a story of cultural richness and culinary innovation. From timeless Moussaka to contemporary Quinoa Paella, you've experienced the evolution of flavors that bridge tradition and modernity.

The inclusion of professional guidance and the importance of seeking expertise have emphasized the collaborative nature of your well-being journey. Like a symphony, where each instrument contributes to harmony, the input of dietitians, fitness trainers, mental health professionals, and healthcare providers plays a vital role in the orchestration of optimal health.

Now, as you conclude this book, envision yourself not at the end but at a new beginning, the beginning of a lifestyle that nourishes your body, delights your senses, and invigorates your spirit. The Mediterranean diet is not a destination; it's a lifelong journey, one where progress is sustained, goals are adapted, and each day is an opportunity to savor the richness of life.

May your future steps echo the dance of longevity, the flavors of well-being, and the symphony of a vibrant and fulfilling existence. "The Mediterranean Diet Decoded" is more than a guide; it's an invitation to a way of living that transcends diets and becomes a legacy of health, joy, and timeless vitality.

Bon voyage on your continued odyssey through the Mediterranean lifestyle, and may each day be seasoned with the richness of well-being.

Cheers to a life decoded, savored, and lived to the fullest!